TOTAL HEALTH WEIGHT LOSS REDEFINED

THE HOLISTIC APPROACH AND ULTIMATE GUIDE ON WEIGHT LOSS AND OBESITY TO ACHIEVE AND MAINTAIN YOUR JOURNEY TO LIFELONG VITALITY THROUGH 7 FACTORS AFFECTING YOUR HEALTH

MICHAEL ERICKSON

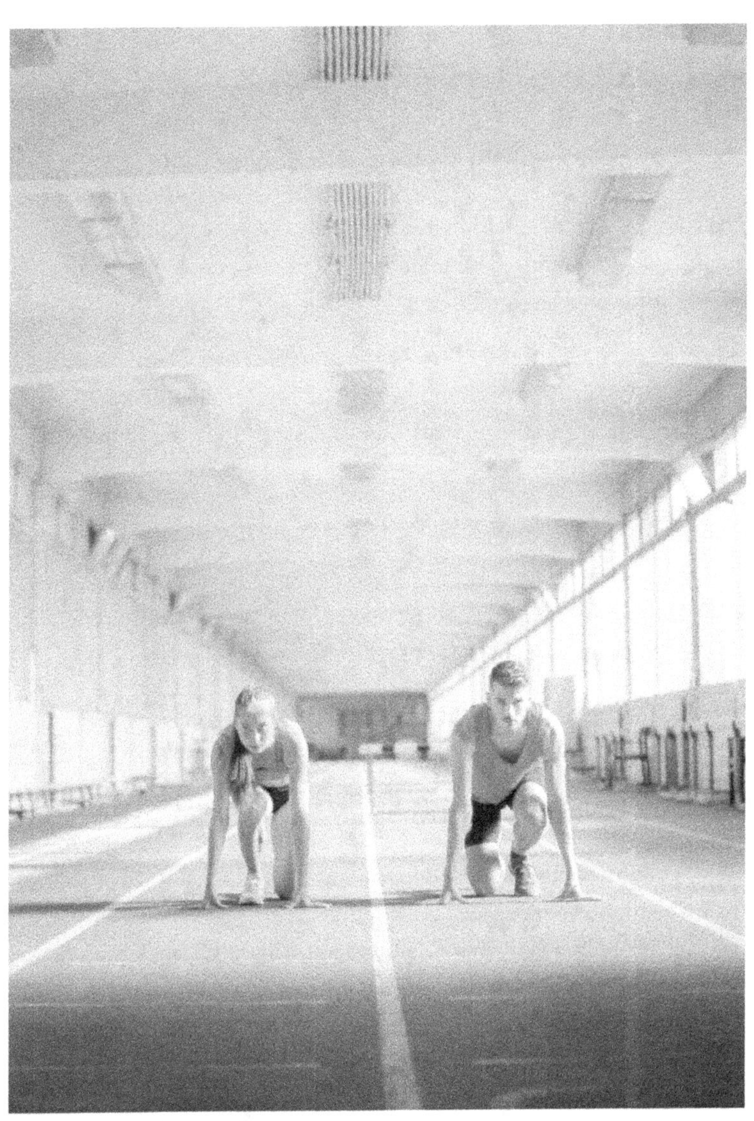

TABLE OF CONTENTS

Introduction   9

1. A CLOSER LOOK AT THE OVERWEIGHT
   EPIDEMIC   17
   Cause   18
   Consequences   19
   Malnutrition and Obesity   20
   Smoking and Obesity   20
   Alcohol and Obesity   22
   Obesity in Older Persons   23
   Obesity in Children and Adolescents   25
   Race, Ethnicity, and Obesity   26
   Genes and Obesity   28
   Obesity and Mental Health   29
   Chapter Summary   30

2. BODY MASS INDEX AND OBESITY   33
   Origins of Adult Obesity   35
   Understanding Obesity   36
   Understanding the Health Risks   41
   Blood-Pressure Measurement   42
   Other Obesity-Related Conditions and
   Diseases   46
   The Effects of Cigarettes and Alcohol   49
   Chapter Summary   52

3. WEIGHT LOSS   55
   Clustering of Lifestyle Risk Factors   56
   The Lies and the Truth of Weight Loss   57
   Medication for Weight Loss   63
   Gastric Bypass Surgery   65
   Gastric Sleeve Surgery   67
   Weight Loss and Exercise   69
   Chapter Summary   78

4. STOP BELIEVING YOU CAN'T   81
    Understanding Metabolism   82
    Increasing Slow Metabolism   85
    Fasting—The Good(-ish) Kind   87
    Losing Weight Too Fast   89
    Healthy Eating on an Ongoing Basis   90
    Metabolic Disorders   94
    Metabolic Syndrome   97
    Weight Cycling   98
    Believing in Yourself   99
    Chapter Summary   101

5. THE MYSTERIES OF DIETS   107
    The History of Dieting   108
    Does Dieting Make You Fat?   109
    Fad Diets   114
    Most Unbelievable Fad Diets   116
    Better Options   119
    Chapter Summary   120

6. SECRETS TO OVERALL HEALTH   123
    Give the Devices a Break   124
    Deep Breathing Exercises   125
    Mindfulness and Awareness   126
    Write It Down   129
    Challenge Yourself   129
    Get the Right Amount of Sleep   130
    Longevity Myths   133
    Chapter Summary   135

7. MANAGING YOUR WEIGHT   137
    What Exactly Is Weight Management?   138
    Exercise for Weight Loss and Management   139
    Why Should You Bother?   148
    Complications   149
    Know Your Stuff   152
    Chapter Summary   154

Conclusion   157
Glossary   167
References   171

INTRODUCTION

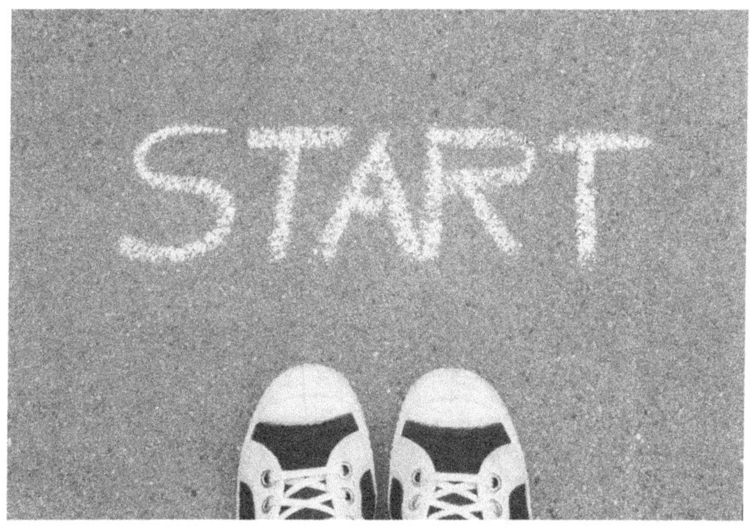

There is no denying that looking after your health is crucially important. We have only one body, and we need to treat it as well as possible. I fully understand the difficulties people face in maintaining a healthy weight. During my childhood, I struggled to lose weight, which led to a number of health implications and emotional consequences.

As an adult, I shed the weight and became healthier in all areas of my life. My total weight reduction was 75 pounds in just 3 months, and I have managed to keep it off. My interest in body health and weight loss was piqued, and, as a result, I have been studying the subject for 25 years.

I decided to write this book because I want to help people who struggle to lose weight or who do lose weight but put it all back on rapidly. I have experienced both sides of the weight-loss fence and I am well-versed in the science behind weight loss and body health. My knowledge is vast, and with knowledge comes power. As I share my knowledge throughout this book, you will be empowered with the know-how to allow you to lose weight, become healthier, and live your best life.

The statistics speak for themselves, and they are nothing short of alarming. A recent study into the mortality rate associated with obesity revealed a startling fact: 1,300 Americans die daily, which works out to almost 500,000 obesity-related deaths each year (Ward et al., 2022). To put this into perspective, 500,000 people would occupy more than 11 Yankee Stadiums.

I could go on quoting statistics, but, as is clear from the above, we have a massive problem. Interestingly and disappointingly, many people have no idea how the body functions. Compare this to a motor vehicle—you might not understand how it works, but you know it needs gas to operate. If it is a petrol engine and you fill it up with diesel, the engine will be destroyed. Similarly, if you keep ingesting food and drinks that do more harm to your body than good, you will destroy it, so to speak.

You need to remember there are both healthy and unhealthy ways to lose weight. We have all heard of celebrities going on crash diets for a few days or a week before a red-carpet event. This is, without a doubt, an incredibly unhealthy method of weight loss, and I will explain the implications. If we were to get technical, I would tell you diets do not work—instead, you need to make a lifestyle adjustment. Going on a diet, even if it is a healthy one, gives the indication the "diet" will come to an end. Then what? Back to your former eating habits.

There is a strong mental element to our relationships with food, and I firmly believe food addiction is a reality for many people. After experiencing a traumatic event, comfort eating can be a coping mechanism. We need to understand these difficulties without judgment, so if you are having issues with food addiction, you will learn it can be beaten. I want you to keep in mind the natural highs and satisfaction that exercise enables—this is the goal.

To be able to adjust our lifestyles, we need to look at the facts of the overweight epidemic and the contributing causes. Thus, we will examine the origins and the conse-quences, during which the contributing factors, such as smoking and drinking, will play a part. We will also discuss other pertinent factors including race, ethnicity, and socioeconomic influences. Mental health has a two-way association with obesity, and you will learn how each influences the other.

The consequences of all this are devastating, and obesity is resulting in major malnutrition. I will explain all of this in Chapter 1 before breaking down the body mass index (BMI) in Chapter 2. A high BMI can indicate high body fatness, while the opposite is true regarding a low BMI. Obesity is influenced by a number of factors, and we will look at prenatal influences as well as adiposity rebound. We will also look at the health risks, including strokes, heart attacks, and diabetes, as well as learn about blood pressure, how it works, and what causes it to reach unhealthy levels. You might have heard all of these terms before, but as you progress through this book, they will become topics of knowledge.

Blood pressure will be explained, including what blood pressure readings actually mean. You will gain an understanding of arrhythmia, cardiomyopathy, and other obesity-related medical conditions. There will be a focus on type 2 diabetes, which is often observed in obese individuals, as well as gallbladder disease, osteoarthritis, and gout.

Two things you will already know are bad habits are alcohol consumption and cigarette smoking, but I am hoping the statistics will help turn you away from them. Clusterings of lifestyle factors and their impact on health, such as the aforesaid smoking and drinking, combined with a lack of fruit intake, will be discussed in Chapter 3.

I will sift through the information to lay bare the lies about weight loss. You will learn not all calories are equal. I want you to appreciate which supplements don't cause weight loss on a large scale, and why skipping breakfast is not always a great idea. The same applies to other health impediments, the biggest of which is overeating. I will explain weight loss and dispel all of its myths. Next is exercise—a vital part of leading a healthy lifestyle—and there are options for everyone, as you'll see.

The logical next step is to examine metabolism—a misunderstood body mechanism. I will explain catabolism and anabolism, and how they make up metabolism as a whole. To further break things down, I will move to explain the basal metabolic rate (BMR) and explain how it is different from the energy used when we exercise. The next point of focus will be healthy eating. I will provide a five-meals-a-day, 7-day recommended eating plan, including breakfast, a morning snack, lunch, an afternoon snack, and dinner. I encourage you to classify the eating plan as a long-term lifestyle change.

There are ways in which a slow metabolism can be increased, but sadly there are some metabolic diseases with no cure. We will focus on both of these subjects and then move on to a more detailed section about metabolic syndrome, characterized by several conditions experienced simultaneously. Then it is on to weight cycling and why it is a bad idea, followed by a bit of motivation to close out Chapter 4.

Chapter 5 kicks off with some thoughts and statistics to back up those thoughts about whether dieting makes you gain weight in the long term. Included is some fascinating information from scientific studies, which sheds light on whether dieting is successful in an overall sense. Fad diets are explained, and you will also receive some tips about healthy choices, mindfulness, and exercise. For a bit of fun, you will learn about some of the craziest fad diets of all time, including the cabbage soup diet and the tapeworm diet. The latter involves ingesting tapeworm eggs under the belief the eggs will hatch, allowing the worms to eat the food you eat and thereby causing you to lose weight.

We can all appreciate eating right and exercising are not the only two components of a healthy lifestyle. Chapter 6 is full of secrets to overall holistic health, including cutting down the time you spend on electronic devices, getting *good* sleep, and practicing deep breathing exercises, as well as detailing everything in a journal and monitoring your progress.

We then will move on to Chapter 7 about weight management. I want to make sure you are not part of the negative statistics. Research shows a very high number of individuals lose weight and then put it all back on and gain more.

Exercise and weight loss go hand in hand, but maintaining your ideal weight once you achieve it takes motivation and focus. Walking just 30 minutes per day for 3 to 4 days a week can keep your weight in check. We will talk about the studies backing this up, and we will look at the benefits of running and cycling for the same purposes. Exercise is not enjoyable for everyone, and for those who want to get it done fast, we will look at intense interval training. There is also information on yoga, Pilates, and swimming for weight maintenance. Don't forget, though: Healthy eating must be a part of your overall health management, in addition to exercise.

You need to avoid a scenario where you get to your ideal weight and then pile the excess back on. On top of the exercise information, we will look at the anatomic and metabolic complications to which obesity is linked, before a section about knowledge on health maintenance. We end with a calorie testing exercise, where you add calories as a test for a certain period after having achieved your weight goals, by which time your knowledge and expertise will be exponentially higher than before you picked up this book. The next step is, of course, action.

There are no quick fixes, and weight-loss gimmicks like the electronic ab belt are just that—gimmicks. Your journey to achieving a healthy weight will involve hard work. There is no way around this fact, but if you can find some inspiration and motivation, then you are a significant distance closer to your ideal weight. My own experiences with weight and health, as mentioned previously, started in my childhood and carried on for many years. I have gained weight, lost it again, put it all back on, and lost it once again. My experiences are ones I have learned from, and, fortunately for you, I can help you learn from my mistakes before you make them yourself. If I had known when I was younger what I know now, my journey to health would have been much quicker. However, I am not angry or resentful. My energy is directed at helping others. I know I can offer help, and I will do my best to extend the offer, but it is up to you to take me up on it. As you continue reading, I believe I can stoke the required inspiration and help you find your motivation. So, let's get into the nitty-gritty, take the very first step, and cross the starting line. Keep your mind open and get ready to turn things around!

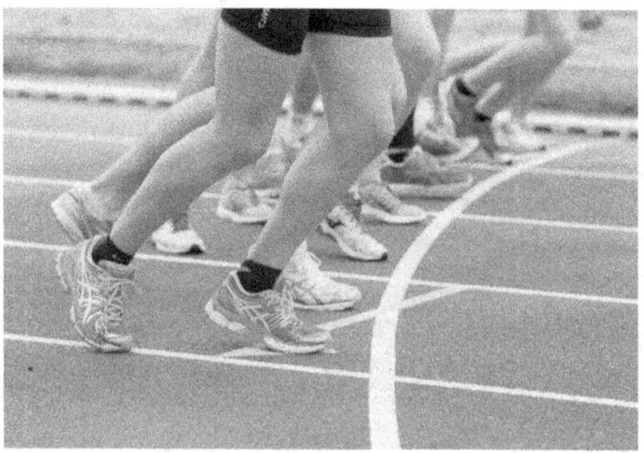

1

A CLOSER LOOK AT THE OVERWEIGHT EPIDEMIC

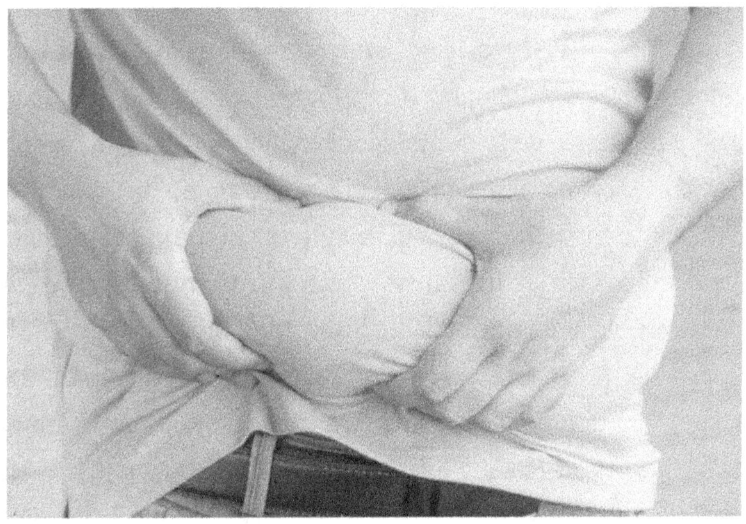

According to statistics, obesity is three times what it was in 1975, with over 650 million obese individuals globally who are over the age of 18 years. In 2020, 39 million children below the age of 5 years were overweight or obese, and most of the world's population lived in countries where more lives were lost to overweight- and obesity-related deaths than to individuals being under-weight (Pu & Huei-Fen, 2023).

Obesity, and being overweight but falling short of obese, are characterized by abnormal or excessive fat accumulation, which may impair health. The term "abnormal" is actually misplaced because being overweight is becoming more common, thus making the correct term "normal," in a sense.

CAUSE

Fundamentally, the cause is simple and logical—too many calories are taken in and not enough calories are burned, causing excess weight. Aside from getting greedier as a human race in general, we are surrounded by energy-dense foods with high sugar and fat content. Combine food intake with the ability to work from home, which a plethora of people are taking advantage of, and the rise of obesity is easily facilitated. Walking to the bus or your car to get yourself to work burns calories, as does getting up from your seat to take a file to a work colleague. Walking around the grocery store is also a calorie killer, but with food delivery, those calories are not being burned at all. You may think the activities mentioned above burn a minimal amount of calories, but if we take walking around for an hour while putting groceries in your cart, you would burn approximately 165 to 220 calories (*Calo-*

ries Burned Shopping, 2020), which is somewhere between two and three slices of pizza. So, if you are having your groceries delivered, the net weight increase you can expect is akin to what a few pizza slices would cause you to gain.

CONSEQUENCES

Noncommunicable diseases—diseases that are not spread through viruses or infections—are associated with obesity and being overweight. Heart attacks and strokes, which fall under "cardiovascular," along with diabetes are among the biggest killers worldwide. Musculoskeletal disorders like arthritis and scoliosis are commonly observed in overweight and obese individuals. Osteoarthritis, which is rapid degeneration of the joints, is highly debilitating and arguably one of the worst musculoskeletal disorders. Certain cancers also pose risks, like liver, kidney, colon, and ovarian, to list a few.

Childhood obesity comes with its own set of consequences, and is responsible for many premature deaths in adulthood. On top of this, obese children often have breathing difficulties, insulin resistance, and hypertension. The psychological impact cannot be ignored, and it is the job of parents to look after the health of their children. As a child, your metabolism *should* naturally be high, so poor and excessive eating is probably more to blame than inactivity, notwithstanding a lot of time being spent indoors using electronic devices.

MALNUTRITION AND OBESITY

Malnutrition is most commonly associated with poverty, but it doesn't actually mean a lack of food. It is possible to eat a lot but not get the nutrients your body requires because of *what* you're eating. In marginalized communities, people eat the cheapest foods, which include bread, maize meal, rice, biscuits, and other carbohydrate-heavy meals. They are getting sustenance, but not by way of healthy eating. The socioeconomic link to obesity and being overweight in these instances is unfortunate, but poverty isn't concerned with health.

On the other hand, if financial circumstances do not limit your choice of food and drink, you can easily become obese while lacking the nutrition required. A diet of energy drinks, greasy foods, and chocolate is not going to give your body what it needs to function optimally.

SMOKING AND OBESITY

There was a time when people believed smoking was healthy or—at the least—posed no health threats. Currently, the data on smoking and linked diseases is abundant. We all know smoking is not good for anyone, but people still do it because it is an addiction. In 2020, the Centers for Disease Control and Prevention did a mass survey among adult smokers. The results showed a total of 480,000 American smokers die every year as a direct consequence of the habit. Furthermore, 16 million smokers in the United States have illnesses as a result of tobacco intake. There was a very small silver lining: Since 2005, the percentage of adult smokers in the US has declined by just over eight percent (Centers for Disease Control and Prevention, 2020).

Like many of the statistics you will encounter in this book, the smoking-related numbers are alarming. But what about smoking to keep thin? This is a theory we need to look in to. Before we do, though, I need to make it clear. Smoking is harmful in every way and provides no benefits whatsoever. Let me remind you, smoking is the number one cause of preventable deaths in the United States.

In any event, it is believed nicotine causes a dip in appetite, and lighting up a cigarette instead of eating is the method of staying thin. Coffee and cigarettes used to be referred to as "the supermodel breakfast," and if you look at how (too) skinny supermodels are, you can understand the reference. The conclusion is you can obviously lose weight by smoking more and eating less. Thus, the weight loss is caused not so much by the actual act of smoking but by the accompanying tactic of minimal food intake.

The next question then becomes, what about overweight and obesity and their connection to smoking? To find the answers, we can look at the results of a 2010 study. The objective of the study was to examine obese and morbidly obese subjects with a view to establishing whether a link between smoking and BMI was present. The participants ranged in age from 18 to 65 and the 1,022 men and women were categorized as nonsmokers, ex-smokers, or smokers. They were also separated in terms of weight, i.e., morbidly obese, obese, overweight, and normal weight as indicated by their BMI readings.

No significant differences in BMI were found in relation to the four weight categories in smokers. There was, however, a trend of more frequent smoking among overweight, obese, and morbidly obese individuals when compared with normal-weight individuals. Another interesting finding was that a morbidly obese individual was two times more likely to become a smoker as opposed to the other categories examined (Chatkin et al., 2010).

ALCOHOL AND OBESITY

When you think of an alcoholic, you may picture someone who is ultrathin, walking the streets, begging for money to buy booze, and who is seriously undernourished. This certainly would not be incorrect, but alcoholism does not discriminate. However, the general mindset is toward a *functional/functioning* alcoholic being more likely to be heavy or obese than an alcoholic who cannot function in society.

But what exactly is a functioning alcoholic? To answer this question, he or she is somebody who can operate day to day, in terms of performing adequately at their job and maintaining good family and social relationships. This type of person is still classified as having alcohol-dependency issues, but is highly likely to believe otherwise.

The point is an out-and-out alcoholic who cannot operate in society will spend money on alcohol before food. Because a functioning alcoholic can hold down a job and maintain a family, their ability, in simple terms, to buy food is alive and well.

Excess alcohol intake or even controlled intake compounds the health risks associated with obesity. Essentially, obesity-linked and alcohol-linked diseases are mashed into one dangerous health risk, potentially causing stroke, heart disease, liver disease, several cancers, high blood pressure, and insulin resistance. We will look at these and more in sections to follow, but for now, we need to recognize the inextricable link between alcohol and obesity.

OBESITY IN OLDER PERSONS

One could take the view of obesity in older people being worse than in those who are younger. You may base this conclusion on the fact older people, in general, are closer to death. The reality is, obesity is always bad, but looking at obesity in adults of mature age can help us educate the younger generation. Let's turn to look at the results of some pertinent studies.

One such study concluded that, over the 30 years preceding the study, the contingent of the obese older adult population in the United States had grown by 50% and obesity across all age groups was continuously on the rise (Patterson et al., 2004). We do have to remember this study was almost 20 years old at the time of publishing this book, but the statistics are nonetheless alarming.

Another study in the same year looked at the obesity crisis from a worldwide perspective, as well as specifically in America. At the time, 7% of the world's population was over 65 years of age. The study predicted this figure would rise to 12% by 2030. The projection for the US was an increase from 12% (35 million) to 20% (71 million) by 2030 (Yan et al., 2004). Adults over the age of 65 years account for 56 million people in the United States. So, with 7 years to go, we may or may not hit the 71 million mark, but we can say without question the US has an aging population. This isn't a massive problem, but what is concerning is the obesity rate in those 65 years old and beyond.

In 2020, approximately 29% of the American population over age 65 was obese. In the same year, the U.S. population of individuals older than 65 was 55 million, meaning roughly 16 million fell into the "over 65 and obese" category—a figure equivalent to three times the entire population of Finland. Yes, a small country, but still an astounding fact (Caplan & Rabe, 2023).

These numbers have got to be an eye opener and we are all obligated to do something about it.

OBESITY IN CHILDREN AND ADOLESCENTS

The Centers for Disease Control and Prevention released a set of statistics derived from data collected between 2017 and 2020. The statistics were for children and adolescents aged between 2 and 19 years, and approximately 14.7 million children and adolescents in this age group were classified as obese. Percentage wise, this amounts to 19.7%. If we break the results down further, obesity prevalence in the 2- to 5-year-old category was recorded at 12.7%; in the 6- to 11-year-old group, the prevalence was 20.7%; and in terms of the 12- to 19-year-olds, 22.2% were affected (Centers for Disease Control and Prevention, 2020).

The upward trend with age certainly tells a story. As is the case with obesity in older persons, the facts and figures are indicative of a major crisis. If you are overweight or obese and (obviously) have a bad diet, it is quite understandable for your children to have the same problem. Inevitably, parents decide what their children eat—not in every single case, but it is the parents who plan the meals, write down the foods to purchase, and buy the groceries, so there is a means of control. However, imposing an unhealthy lifestyle on someone who doesn't have a great amount of power to choose is something parents should seek to eliminate.

A multitude of studies have produced conclusive evidence showing children with obese or overweight parents are more likely to become overweight or obese themselves. One of the leading and most recent sets of studies found a child is 1.97 times more likely to become overweight or obese if one or both of their parents is overweight or obese, when compared to a child with two parents of healthy weight (Lee et al., 2022).

If we look at this practically, adult obesity is on the rise; this means, as per the "1.97 times" finding, childhood obesity must also be on the rise. One would be hesitant to say this is genetic, but it cannot be argued genes do not have an impact at all. Let's examine this a bit more.

RACE, ETHNICITY, AND OBESITY

These factors are linked to socioeconomic influences because of the prevalence of marginalized communities in the United States. There are mild genetic considerations, but the biggest link is poverty. Unfortunately, we are not doing enough to assist those who are disadvantaged and face consequences of circumstance. In 2021, the Annie. E Casey Foundation found children of color experienced more situations of poverty than their White counterparts. Statistically, in the US, 28% of Black, 25% of American Indian, and 23% of Latino children are likely to be brought up in poor households, as opposed to the figures for White and Pacific Island children, being 10% and 9% respectively (Annie E. Casey Foundation, 2021).

Looking at those percentages, it is easy to understand that when the money available for food is limited, the trend is to buy the cheapest possible foods. Those foods are the types high in carbohydrates, sugar, and fat, so the result is increased obesity in these marginalized communities. Here, the solution is near impossible until social services improve their care of the disadvantaged. On top of grants and welfare, there needs to be education across the board, part of which should encompass health education.

The Centers for Disease Control and Prevention (2022) provides the following data on obesity among the marginalized:

- Hispanic youth: 22.4%
- Non-Hispanic Black youth: 20.2%
- Non-Hispanic White youth: 14.1%
- Non-Hispanic Asian youth: 8.6%

The crux of the matter is obesity in this particular category is on the rise, just like it is in every other category;

however, the really sad part is that in *this* category the solution is much less achievable than in the others.

GENES AND OBESITY

The merging of the two above terms results in a constructed term, i.e., "obesogenic." Social factors rather than actual genetics make up obesogenic environments, which are defined as "the sum of influences that surroundings, opportunities, or conditions of life have on promoting obesity in individuals or a population" (Swinburn et al., 1999). Those influences would include proximity to grocery stores as opposed to fast food outlets. If you can walk half a mile to get a takeaway, as opposed to taking a bus 5 miles to get groceries, the former option is both cheaper and more convenient. If your surroundings do not promote exercise, you are less likely to exercise than if there was a local focus on exercise. Lack of education is another strong factor, as in these cases food science is probably not a contributing factor to your decision on what to eat.

In terms of actual genes passed down from family member to family member, we will address this in detail in further chapters. But, briefly, genetics can directly cause obesity in specific disorders. Multiple gene combinations may have an influence, but outside factors such as overeating and no exercise are also needed as contributors for an individual to become obese.

OBESITY AND MENTAL HEALTH

Mental health has been in the spotlight in terms of the effects of social media on teenagers and young adults. There is no denying that depression is on the rise, and, in addition to social media, obesity has a strong link with both anxiety and depression. There is understandably a fair amount of embarrassment felt by many overweight and obese individuals, as well as the reality of being teased and picked on. These are all contributors to poor mental health, which cannot be completely separated from physical health.

A 2006 study observed a 25% increase in the chances of mood and anxiety disorders associated with obesity. Substance use disorders as a result of obesity were also pinned at approximately 25%. Moreover, social circumstances, cultural oppression, and belonging to either a minority or majority group were all found to have influence over obesity and mood and anxiety disorders (Simon et al., 2006).

Considering the study was conducted approximately 17 years ago, it would not be remiss to presume those statistics are substantially higher in 2023. At the end of the day we are all people and our differences need to be ignored if we want to help each other out of the circumstances that continue to perpetuate poor health.

The reverse also applies, i.e., mental health disorders can lead to obesity, the link being eating and drinking as a form of self-medication. People who are depressed have serotonin deficiencies, which also affect sleep patterns and can result in food consumption as a coping mechanism. A lack of desire to exercise is often a symptom of depression and, when overeating and excessive drinking are added into the mix, the propensity for obesity increases substantially.

CHAPTER SUMMARY

If you take only one thing from this chapter—and I know you know this—it should be that obesity is a growing problem, and we need to take collective responsibility to address it. The simplicity of the concept of "fewer calories ingested than burned" does not mean the situation can be changed in a simple way. However, by starting with this fundamental concept, we can put in the work needed.

It goes without saying: The consequences are dire due to a multitude of factors. Obesity is the result of malnutrition and can be worsened by combining smoking and excessive drinking. This combination compounds health risks that are prevalent across the age spectrum. Race and ethnicity influence obesity, as they are tied to socioeconomic disadvantages: less money = more unhealthy foods. Obesity can be a contributing factor to anxiety, depression, and other mental health conditions. The reverse is also prevalent, as depressed individuals with a lack of motivation to exercise also self-medicate with excessive eating and drinking.

So, to take stock, we now know the specifics of the overweight and obese epidemic, and we are ready to look closely at the operation of our bodies in consideration of BMI.

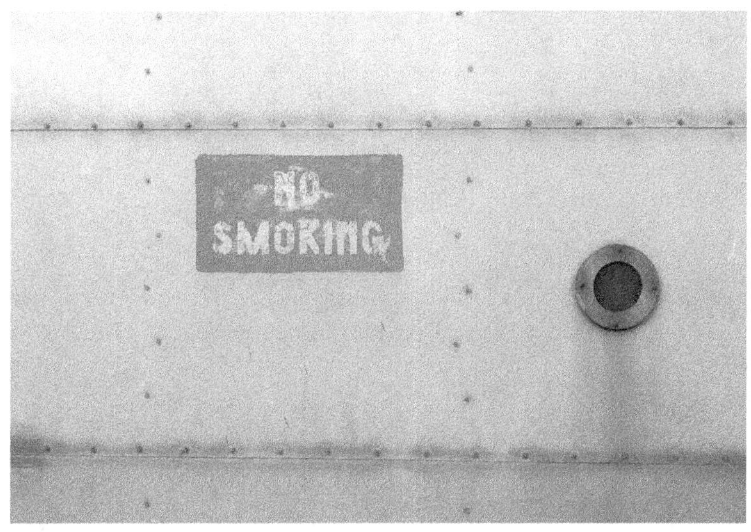

2

BODY MASS INDEX AND OBESITY

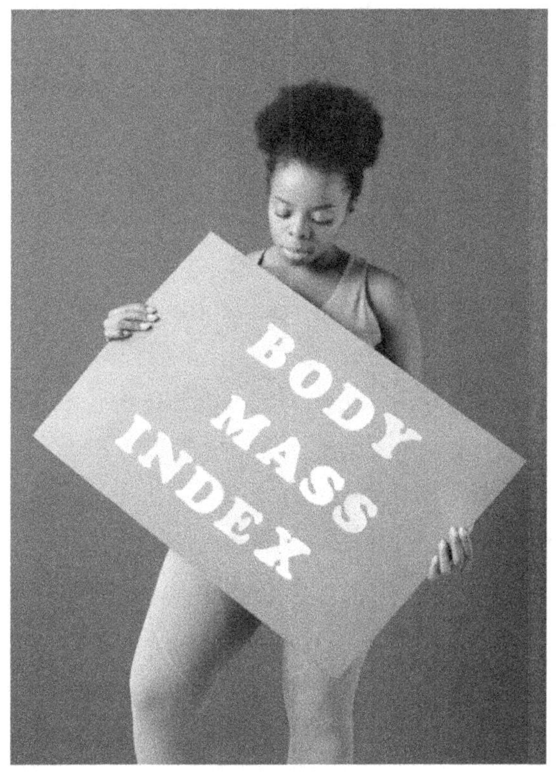

You may have heard the term BMI—which you will remember from earlier in this book means body mass index—but perhaps you do not know quite what it is. Well, BMI takes your weight and divides it by your height squared. The weight measurements are done in kilograms and the height measurements in meters and centimeters. Although establishing BMI is not terribly difficult, it does not actually diagnose health problems. For this reason, BMI is an indicator of the extent of the possibility of having health issues or developing them. This means BMI cannot be used to label an individual as "fat" or "unhealthy"; however, we can draw strong inferences from our BMI. In fact, BMI was developed as a risk indicator. The word "indicator" is important because BMI results are not like a blood test with a definite finding, but rather are an indicator of poor health.

Research into what would later be termed BMI was kicked off by American physiologist Ancel Keys in Minnesota in 1947. The motivation for his research was extensive and he aimed to uncover the reasons for what appeared to be a puzzling increase in the deaths of many seemingly healthy middle-aged Minnesota men. In 1958, Keys created the *Seven Countries Study*, which was a long-term research project on the relationship between one's diet and coronary heart disease. Ancel Keys' study (Keys, 1958) is considered to be the most significant of his career and involved a large variety of subjects from the United

States, Greece, Italy, Spain, South African, Japan, and Finland.

Thanks to Keys, and various of his successors, BMI has become a comprehensive measure using height and weight to work out if your weight is healthy or not. For example, a 1.75 meter tall, 70 kilogram adult will have a BMI of 22.9 (70 divided by 1.75 squared). A BMI of 22.9 sits squarely in the middle of the ideal range for adults, which is 18.5 to 24.9. If your BMI falls below 18.5 you are considered underweight, whereas a BMI between 25 and 29.9 makes you overweight. The most concerning category, health wise, is "obese," and anyone with a BMI of over 30 is considered obese. The risk of cardiovascular disease then becomes very real. If you know your height and weight, you will be able to plot your BMI using one of the many BMI calculators online—simply type "BMI calculator" into your preferred search engine.

ORIGINS OF ADULT OBESITY

I am certain you have heard the term "big boned," often used as an explanation for people who have a proclivity to put on weight or who are overweight. Well, this is an urban legend, which means it is not an excuse (although we should not be looking for excuses in the first place). Our skeletons obviously weigh something, but are generally in proportion to our size. As an example, a man weighing 90 kilograms would have a skeleton totaling about 10 to 14 kilograms, which translates into roughly 12% to 15% of his total body weight. If you were to pick out an equivalent example for a woman, the percentage would translate into a skeletal weight of somewhere between 8 and 11 kilograms (De Brabandere, 2017).

UNDERSTANDING OBESITY

There is an argument for obesity being a disease, but a counterargument for obesity being self-inflicted. Both positions have their merits, but if obesity is indeed a disease, the cure is to lose weight. One could say the same for alcoholism, which can be cured by drinking less alcohol. Another school of thought regards obesity as an addiction—or, alternatively, as the result of an addiction. Consider gambling—the addiction is the action of gambling, and the result is loss of money. It then follows that food is the actual addiction when it comes to being overweight or obese, which is the *result* of the addiction.

Many people in this world eat for sustenance and not for taste. I am not saying those people don't enjoy the taste of food, and just eat it because their body requires nutrition. However, they see food in a different way. We also have to think about addictive personalities. Some people seem to be less able to resist the urge to indulge, and I am sure you have all been offered a snack before and had to say no because you knew if you had one thing to eat, then the floodgates would open and you would be unable to resist having more. This was certainly the case for me when I was at my unhealthiest and heaviest.

A University of Michigan study revealed one in eight Americans over the age of 50 displays signs of food addiction. The study was based on an extensive poll, which found highly processed foods to be particularly addictive. The poll also took into account physical and mental health. Regarding the former, 32% of women reported fair or poor physical health, as did 14% of men. In terms of the latter, 45% of women considered their mental health to be fair or poor. The male contingent who reported fair to poor mental health represented 23% of participants (Gearhardt et al, 2023).

These statistics are incredibly important. I can't stress this enough, and in the same breath I am hoping readers of this book will be shocked, and that such shock will inspire the need to lose weight and get healthy. Yes, it is a harsh attitude, but the endemic obesity problem is a harsh reality!

As I mentioned previously, the formula is simple: calories in versus calories burned. But there are some social and environmental factors that could be at play, which have been studied comprehensively. Let's take a look at these factors, but please remember: At the end of the day, it is up to the individual to change, whether or not any factors whatsoever are at play.

Prenatal Factors

The thinking here is there are signs you can look for in an expectant mother that may lend themselves to future weight issues for the child. One of the earliest studies in this area looked at Dutch women during the famine in German-occupied The Netherlands in World War II and concluded, "progeny (offspring) of survivors of the famine demonstrated a higher prevalence of obesity and diabetes" (Ravelli et al., 1976).

As happens with research, Ravelli's 1976 study was questioned in the early 1990s. However, studies in future years indicated Ravelli's findings had been correct. One such study concluded, "malnutrition, especially in the first two trimesters, can result in complications associated with obesity" (Stanner et al., 1997).

A later study examined the developmental origins of adult health and disease, and its findings became known as the Developmental Origins of Health and Disease (DOHaD) hypothesis, which states the following: "Exposure to an unfavorable environment during development (either in utero or in the early postnatal period) programmes changes in fetal or neonatal development such that the individual is then at greater risk of developing adulthood disease" (Armitage et al., 2008).

The science isn't conclusive enough to pin obesity directly to these factors, and in fact the DOHaD study stated further: "There is no doubt much of the trending rise in obesity can be attributed to lifestyle factors such as the excess consumption of energy-dense foods and the decline in physical activity (Armitage et al., 2008).

Adiposity Rebound

"Adiposity" refers to having too much fatty tissue in your body. Fatty tissue naturally grows until about the age of 1 year, then progressively declines until approximately 5 to 7 years old. "Rebound" indicates an increase in BMI and fat after the decline.

While adiposity rebound has been studied in some detail, there have been different conclusions. It was first thought that children who experience the rebound at an earlier stage had three to six times more chance of an elevated BMI in later life than other children (Aronoff et al., 2022).

A prominent study into adiposity rebound tasked itself with examining all available scientific publications on the subject. After doing so, the situation remained unclear in terms of adiposity rebound age and how critical it is for later obesity development. Researchers did conclude that adiposity rebound *could* be a statistical indicator of future obesity. This conclusion was based on the link between early adiposity and maturing at a faster rate, which do appear to indicate higher chances of developing obesity (Cameron & Demerath, 2002).

The study is important, but you could argue lifestyle factors have a bigger influence over obesity, and resigning yourself to becoming obese because of early adiposity rebound is giving up on health before even giving it a chance.

Adolescence

There is a lack of research and probably not enough data to make any concrete conclusion, but it is estimated that 30% of adult obesity begins during childhood. Furthermore, 70% of adult obesity begins during adolescence (adolescence is considered as age range 10 to 19 years; technically, until 19 you are still a child).

These estimations don't change the indisputable fact we are experiencing an obesity crisis, and, of course, the usual risks of obesity-related diseases remain present, even at a young age.

Other Factors

If we were to get technical, we could break down a whole bunch of factors and examine them. Things like genetics, race, ethnicity, and gender may have influences on obesity, whether in children, adolescents, or adults, but we don't want to delve too deeply into the science, which focuses on reasons or origins. Rather, we want to solve the problem by understanding the actual health risks that don't change.

UNDERSTANDING THE HEALTH RISKS

Obesity is likely to lead to high blood pressure, also called hypertension, which can be the catalyst of adverse heart health. Think of your cardiovascular system as a hosepipe snaking around in a garden. The water circulates through the pipe, just as blood moves through the cardiovascular/circulatory system through a complex set of arteries. The blood contains oxygen, in addition to electrolytes, vitamins and nutrients, which nourish organs and tissues. Another function of the blood flow is to collect toxins, which we then clear through our liver and kidneys. It also provides a defense against tissue damage and essentially looks after the well-being of the body.

The flow of your blood puts pressure on your arteries, and, as you can imagine, too much pressure is not a good thing. Although the heart creates the initial surge of pressure, your arteries maintain the pressure required to pump the blood around the body. If your blood pressure is high, then the elasticity of your arteries is reduced, and as those arteries become narrower, too little blood flows through them.

BLOOD-PRESSURE MEASUREMENT

Normal or "acceptable" blood pressure levels are below 120 over 80, but what does this actually mean? The first number (120) is the measurement of the pressure in your arteries created by your heartbeat, known as systolic blood pressure. The second number is the diastolic blood pressure, which is the pressure on your arteries in between your heartbeats.

Diagnosing high blood pressure varies from medical care provider to medical care provider. There is no definitive agreement as to what constitutes high blood pressure, but the two ranges that are most recognized as indicative of concerningly high blood pressure are 140 over 90 or 130 over 80. Definitive agreement is, however, present on the medical implications high blood pressure can bring with it, and the consequences can be dire.

Heart Disease

Under the umbrella of heart disease you get arrhythmia, cardiomyopathy, coronary heart disease, and heart failure.

Arrhythmia

Our hearts beat in time with a specific rhythm, but when an alternative rhythm is present, whether it is your heart slowing down, speeding up, or quivering, the sensation most often passes quickly. In most cases there is nothing to worry about, but on occasion (in the context of heart disease numbers) you could experience effects on your blood flow, which can be dangerous.

Cardiomyopathy

This refers to an abnormal heart muscle that struggles to effectively pump blood through your cardiovascular system. Over time, if left untreated, cardiomyopathy can cause heart failure. There are three main types of cardiomyopathy, namely restrictive, diluted, and hypertrophic heart failure. Unfortunately symptoms may only present themselves some time after cardiomyopathy arises. The most common symptoms are dizziness, a feeling of pressure on the chest, abdominal bloating, extreme fatigue, and a persistent cough that worsens when lying down.

Coronary Heart Disease

Coronary heart disease is when fatty deposits build up in the coronary arteries, which limit or constrict blood flow to the heart. Your heart muscle starts dying because it is not getting enough blood, and often a heart attack is the result, which in many cases becomes the indicator of the presence of coronary heart disease.

Heart Failure

Most cases of heart failure are the result of coronary artery disease and heart attacks. It is not a case of your heart ceasing to work, but rather your heart expanding in size in an effort to pump faster and cause more blood to flow through the clogged arteries. The result is weakening of the heart muscle, which leads to less blood flow, meaning your heart has attempted or is attempting to rescue the situation by putting strain on itself. Symptoms of heart failure include wheezing, swollen ankles and feet, irregular or rapid heartbeat, wheezing, nausea, and lack of appetite.

Further Heart Health Issues

I am sure a heart attack would be considered by most to be a wake-up call and an instigator of taking steps toward improving your health, but it would be much better not to get to this point at all. Of course, a heart attack is not the only way your body might tell you the time has come to make a change, or, in extreme cases, does not allow you that choice. You have to change or your body will suffer the consequences.

Sudden Cardiac Death

When the heart's electrical system causes irregular and/or dangerously fast beats, its chambers will start to quiver. In this scenario a defibrillator is essentially the only method of regulating your heartbeat, otherwise you will probably die in under 5 minutes.

Heart Attack

As everyone knows, a heart attack can easily result in death, but if treated soon after it begins then death can be prevented. A heart attack happens when the blood clots and cannot get through the arteries. Blood supply to the heart becomes cut off, meaning no oxygen reaches the heart. Most often heart attacks are sudden, but on occasion the symptoms can be recurring but very mild, until the attack actually takes place. In terms of mildness of the symptoms, alarm bells may not be raised if discomfort is not hugely significant. This is why heart attacks can seem sudden, but if you are overweight or obese, then even mild symptoms should provoke a visit to the doctor. By way of an example, shortness of breath can be a sign of a heart attack that can appear on its own. Someone who is asthmatic would have experienced shortness of breath many times, and may write it off to something asthma related, not realizing it is a precursor to a heart attack. Other symptoms include chest pain and discomfort in the arms, neck, jaw, back, or stomach, as well as cold sweats and possible nausea.

Stroke

In the case of a stroke, the arteries that carry oxygen to the brain burst because they are blocked significantly, and often completely. Because our brain cells die during a stroke, speech and basic movement can be affected negatively. Death is also a possibility, but do remember a stroke and a heart attack are not the same thing. A stroke is brain related and a heart attack is clearly heart related, but both are caused by high blood pressure.

OTHER OBESITY-RELATED CONDITIONS AND DISEASES

The heart is not the only organ at risk of malfunctioning due to the implications of being overweight or obese. There are many other related conditions, which, if unmanaged, can become fatal. Let me remind you, the conditions we are about to address can be deadly if you do not make a lifestyle change.

Type 2 Diabetes

People affected by obesity are about six times more likely to have high blood sugar, otherwise known as high blood glucose (WebMD Editorial Contributors, 2021). Type 2 diabetes is a long-term condition where too much sugar is circulating in the blood, and is mainly associated with older adults. However, with the rise of obesity levels in children, type 2 diabetes has been observed in increasing numbers in younger people. It is not curable, but losing weight, eating better, and exercising can manage the condition. Medication and insulin therapy are available in terms of management, but, obviously, a healthy lifestyle could be preventative in the first place.

Cancer

Over 684,000 cancer deaths annually in the United States are obesity related (Centers for Disease Control and Prevention, 2020). As alarming as this figure is, getting into shape will seriously decrease the possibility of becoming part of the statistics. Colon, breast, endometrium, esophagus, and kidney cancer are all linked to obesity. Treatments like chemotherapy and radiation are generally better handled by people of normal weight than individuals who are overweight or obese.

Gallbladder Disease

Your gallbladder is found under the kidneys. It releases bile into your small intestine as a means of digestion assistance. Gallstones may form in your gallbladder; these are hardened bits of digestive fluid and can result in intense and persistent pain. If untreated, or in very severe cases, gallstones can lead to death, but surgery is known to clear gallstones and has proven to be an effective and relatively straightforward operation. In addition to obesity, losing weight too fast can also result in gallstones. Gallbladder disease is experienced by about 20% of healthy adults. With such a high rate of adult gallbladder disease among *healthy* individuals, you can imagine how the risks increase for overweight and obese adults.

Osteoarthritis

To use a simple analogy, osteoarthritis is wear and tear on your joints. The cartilage, which works as cushioning between joints, is worn away. Logically, excess weight places more pressure on your joints, so the cartilage wears away faster. Unfortunately, there is no cure. However, weight loss reduces the pressure imposed on the joints and can result in a reduction in the pain associated with osteoarthritis. Short-term relief from the pain associated with osteoarthritis can be sought through painkillers and anti-inflammatory drugs. Heating and cooling the area, as well as massage, are also methods for temporary respite. Prevention is often better than cure, and if you can lose weight, you are most definitely increasing your chances of preventing the development of osteoarthritis. Maintaining a generally healthy lifestyle, on top of first losing the weight, is also very important in terms of prevention.

Gout

Too much uric acid in your blood can cause crystallization in the joints, or gout, which is very painful. It is often accompanied by swelling around the affected joints. Gout is common in obese individuals and is actually a type of arthritis. Again, excess weight on the joints can worsen the condition. Similarly to osteoarthritis, temporary relief from gout can be achieved via pharmaceutical drugs, usually containing sodium. Also, adjusting your lifestyle factors can help to prevent the onset of gout. Just like osteoarthritis, it is much better to prevent gout by losing weight and increasing healthy habits.

Sleep Apnea

More than 45% of obese adults experience serious cases of sleep apnea. Sleep apnea is the narrowing of the airway during sleep, which causes brief periods where no breaths are taken in at all. Snoring is very common, as well as gasping in the way you would after being kept underwater by a wave. Sleep apnea often disrupts proper sleep, resulting in excessive tiredness during the day. It also makes the chances of stroke and various heart diseases much higher.

THE EFFECTS OF CIGARETTES AND ALCOHOL

Previously, we looked at the links between cigarettes and weight, in addition to alcohol and weight. What follows is a short section on the direct diseases linked to both smoking and excessive drinking.

Everyone knows cigarettes have zero health benefits, but lung cancer statistics suggest people don't care. Excessive alcohol use has devastating effects on the body and on health in general. When combined with being overweight or obese, cigarettes and alcohol have an even greater negative impact.

Cigarettes

The effects of cigarettes compound the chances of heart disease, stroke, and diabetes. Being a smoker who is also obese means you are putting yourself in danger by eating too much and enjoying cigarettes—and remember, you shouldn't be enjoying them! Other diseases associated with smoking are as follows:

- cancer (throat, lung, or other)
- lung diseases
- emphysema
- chronic bronchitis
- tuberculosis
- eye diseases
- rheumatoid arthritis

As of 2021, more than 16 million Americans were living with a disease caused by smoking. For every person who dies because of smoking, at least 30 people live with a serious smoking-related illness (Centers for Disease Control and Prevention, 2021).

Alcohol

In excessive amounts, alcohol can be a major factor in obesity and the inability (or lack of effort) to lose weight. Other than preventing your body from losing fat, alcohol is high in kilojoules, often makes you hungry, and assists in creating cravings for salt-heavy and greasy foods. Heavy and/or high-risk drinking refers to individuals who have more than three drinks on any one day or more than seven drinks averaged out over a week for women and men older than age 65. For men and women under 65, the mark is more than four drinks on any one day or more than 14 drinks averaged out over a week (Mayo Clinic Staff, 2021).

Just as cigarettes increase the chances of diseases even more than usual in overweight and obese individuals, alcohol follows suit. Here are some dangers associated with heavy drinking:

- certain cancers, including breast cancer and cancers of the mouth, throat, esophagus, and liver
- persistent pancreatic infections
- pancreatitis
- dying suddenly if you already have cardiovascular disease
- alcoholic cardiomyopathy, which, in simple terms, is heart muscle damage leading to heart failure
- stroke
- high blood pressure
- liver disease

The best option is to give up alcohol altogether in your pursuit of health. Otherwise, it is imperative to drink at levels that are not threatening to your health.

CHAPTER SUMMARY

BMI, or body mass index, can be an indicator of an individual's propensity to health problems and helps us categorize weight groups. Food addiction, however, leads to a disregard for BMI and its indicators because often people don't care—another thing that needs to change. It is interesting to note the prenatal influences on future obesity and weight management. Another influence we looked at was adiposity, which is a build-up of fatty tissue with serious health consequences. I am not going to repeat every health risk, but please remember the importance of blood-pressure measurements and their associations with the many heart diseases leading to heart attacks, sudden cardiac death, and strokes. The consequences of cigarettes and alcohol and subsequent conditions include lung disease, emphysema, tuberculosis, liver disease, and certain cancers, among others.

Leaving everything else aside, because there are aspects of this chapter where people's opinions may differ, the resounding conclusion is we need to look after our health. Now we have a deeper understanding of obesity and its associated health risks, it is time to turn to the practicalities of losing weight and hence improving health. A quick interesting weight loss fact before we move on: The most weight lost in a lifetime by a man is 2,268 kg (5,000 lb; 357 st; 2.2 tonnes), achieved by Michael Hebranko (Seddon, 2012).

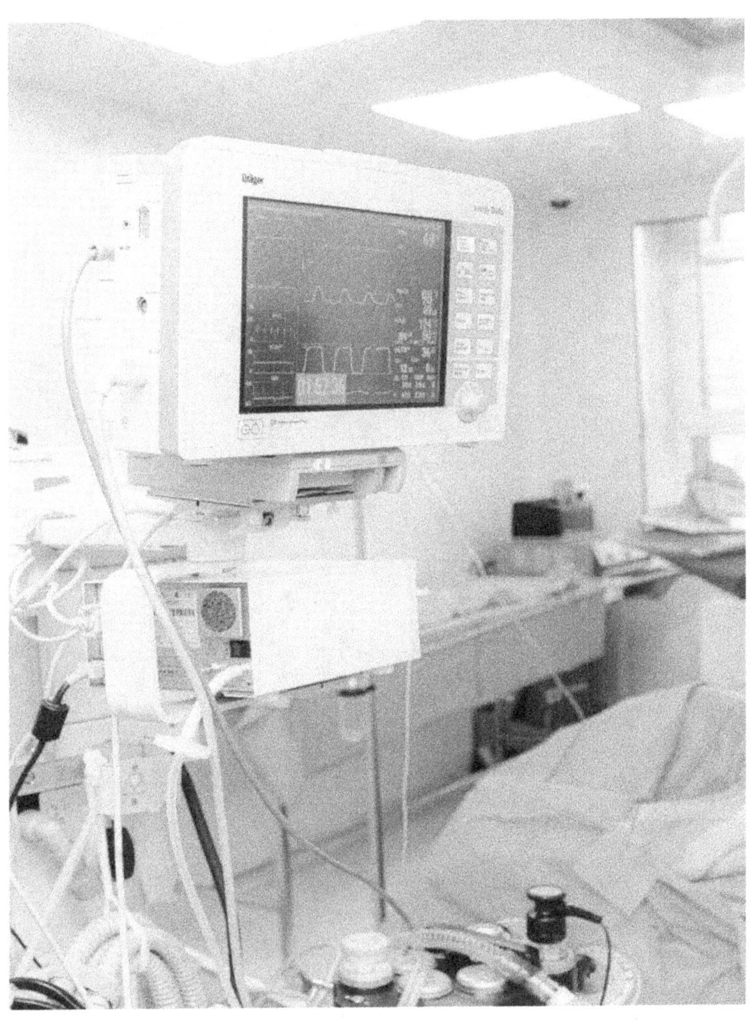

3

WEIGHT LOSS

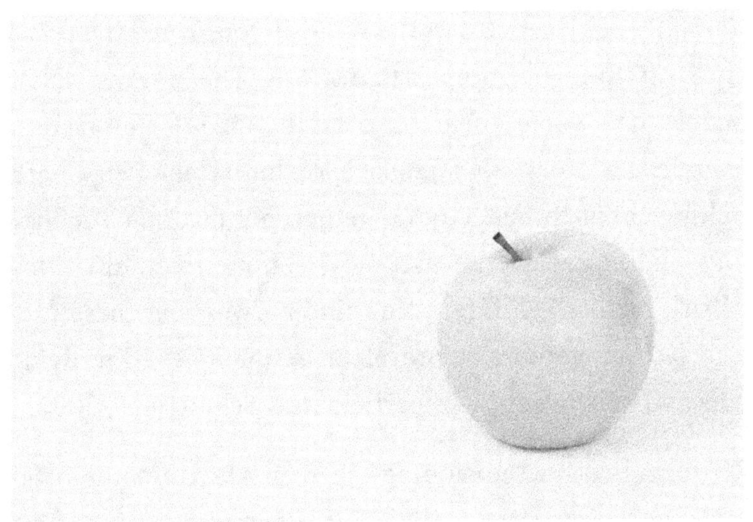

There is more than one lifestyle risk factor associated with weight loss, as you know. These risk factors can manifest both mentally and physically. When several of the risk factors are combined, it is called a clustering of lifestyle risk factors. Many have tried to lose weight. Many have failed. Many have succeeded. Many have done both. A clustering of lifestyle risk factors can be a difficult set of habits to cull. Let's break this down a little further by looking at a study focusing on clustering in adults.

CLUSTERING OF LIFESTYLE RISK FACTORS

The study involved 16,789 men and women aged between 20 and 59. The makeup of the cluster in this case specifically involved smoking, excessive alcohol intake, lack of exercise, and lack of vegetable and fruit intake. It was found that at least 20% of the subjects confirmed the presence of three or more risk factors. This means 3,558 people had some form of combination of the factors examined. It doesn't *sound* like a lot, but remember we are talking about three factors together, not just one. Alcohol and smoking were the two most common combinations of risk factors. An interesting finding was that these two risk factors were more prevalent in unemployed individuals and poorly educated participants (Schuit et al., 2002).

To speculate on the findings in relation to unemployed and poorly educated individuals, unemployment can be mentally taxing, and indulging in risk factors could be more of a misguided self-medication tactic. Having limited education probably limits a person's cognition to appreciate risk factors. After all, between 1930 and 1950, doctors actually *recommended* smoking (Klara, 2015). Yes, this was a long time ago, but take an individual today who does not have a high school diploma compared with a doctor from the mid-20th century.

The study did not examine weight specifically. However, a "healthy weight" does not indicate complete body health. There are plenty of people who smoke, drink, and exercise and think they are remedying the harm of alcohol and cigarettes by exercising. Being active is important, but poisoning your body, even if you are active, does not mean you cannot still have high blood pressure and thus high risks of the associated conditions. We should not be lying to ourselves about this, or ignoring it, so let's delve into some truths about weight loss.

THE LIES AND THE TRUTH OF WEIGHT LOSS

There is a lot of information out there about weight loss. Something pertinent to remember is supplement manufacturers want to sell supplements, personal trainers want clients, and pharmaceutical companies want to make money off weight-loss products. I am not making accusations, but often money is the motivator instead of actually helping people. In addition, there are myths out there, some of which we do not even know the origin of. Others have been propagated by science, and with the advent of better technology and methods of research, previous studies have been proven wrong.

All Calories Are Equal

A calorie is a calorie is a calorie? Not quite. All calories have the same energy content, but not all calories have the same effect on your body. Look at it like distance measurements—a kilometer is always a kilometer, but uphills and downhills will have different effects depending on which way you are walking. The point is, certain things that are always the same do not always cause the same result.

Different foods pass through different pathways as your body metabolizes them. Replacing carbohydrates and fatty foods with protein will boost your metabolism and reduce any cravings. You will not become as hungry as you would if you only ate carbs and fat, plus protein works as a weight-regulating hormone optimizer.

Carbohydrates Make You Fat

Obviously, if you eat pizza every day and do no exercise, you will get fat. If you keep your carb consumption low and your protein consumption high, you will lose weight. It is more about the amount eaten than what you eat, and don't forget the human race has been eating carbs for a very long time. Fad diets, which we will touch on later, are often anti-carb, but we have to remember a fad is not always a good thing.

Weight Loss Moves in One Direction

Body weight fluctuates due to several reasons, so even if you give up your vices, begin to eat a healthy diet, and start an exercise regime, your weight may fluctuate. Water retention and carrying more food than usual in your digestive system have an influence on weight. As long as the general direction is down, with a few upward blips, then you are doing a good job. If you have been successful in losing weight in the past, you will know sometimes you just feel "thinner" than other times. Bloating can have an effect, otherwise daily activity may have an influence on the way your body feels.

You Must Eat Breakfast if You Want to Lose Weight

This is an instance where earlier studies have been proved wrong by later studies as technology and methods improved. It was initially thought people who don't eat breakfast tend to weigh more than those who have breakfast every day. There was a theory that a contributing factor is people who eat breakfast are likely to also engage in further healthy habits. The amount you eat for breakfast or during any meal will also have an impact. Without a doubt, the best approach is to eat when you're hungry and stop eating when you are full—or, ideally, just before you are full (Horikawa et al., 2011).

Supplements Cause Weight Loss

It is quite rare for supplements to be studied sufficiently for their claims to be backed up with actual evidence. The reason for this is that many scientists don't consider supplements as worthy of extensive study. A handful of supplements have a very small effect on weight loss, but for the most part, the manufacturers are only concerned with profits. Some believe there is a placebo effect, which helps with weight loss. Having said this, supplements will often accompany better eating and exercise, which disguise the lack of effect of the supplements. Basically, in such cases, the eating and the exercise are doing the job, while the supplements are a waste of money.

Eating Fat Makes You Fat

Interestingly, fat has approximately double the calories per gram than carbohydrates. Eating a high-fat, low-carb diet can, and has been shown to, aid weight loss quite significantly. Fat provided by junk food is another story, and excess junk food will undoubtedly cause weight gain. Our body's functionality depends on many things, one of which is healthy fats.

Fast Food Is Always Fattening

Traditionally, the term "fast food" is associated with fatty, greasy, processed food that has little health benefit but tastes delicious. These days there are far more healthy options at fast food and takeaway outlets, which are just as delicious but way kinder to your body. A chicken wrap with lettuce, cheese, and tomato is obviously better than a fried chicken burger with french fries.

Diet Foods Make You Lose Weight

Money over truth should be the motto of many food producers and restaurants. Certain foods are marketed as "diet foods," or foods that improve health or have X, Y, and Z health properties, but in reality, it just is not true. Just because the advert, the packaging, or the salesperson tells you something is healthy, it may not be true—I would advise some skepticism.

Diets Work

I mentioned crash diets earlier, especially in the case of celebrities who engage in these diets with the goal of looking slim at red-carpet events. However, I did not go into the specifics of the different crash diets. The thing is, they do work in the short term, but overall a crash diet does not work on a long-term basis. For example, a popular fast weight-loss diet is the grape diet. It involves eating only grapes and drinking only grape juice for 5 days, along with an intense exercise regime. Extreme diets like this are very unhealthy, and any health professional would issue a severe warning not to engage. These methods do not have any sustainability, and nor do diets claimed to be "healthier." The name of the game is lifestyle change in all areas requiring such change, in a sustainable manner that promotes living your healthiest life.

Obese Means Unhealthy, and Slim Means Healthy

Many fit and slim people die of heart attacks, are crippled by strokes, or have type 2 diabetes. Obesity is associated way more with poor health than being thin, but it is not the case for every overweight person to be completely unhealthy and for every slim person to be completely healthy. If you are smoking a pack of cigarettes a day and taking in minimal food, the chances your health is good are pretty slim. Also, a number of heavy drinkers seem to have suppressed appetites or just prefer to drink than to eat, giving the illusion they are healthy.

Getting Over Obesity Is ONLY About Willpower

In the previous chapter, we looked at factors that influence obesity, some of which are out of our control. One I didn't mention is the side effects of medication. Certain medications for depression make patients more likely to put on weight. Then there are conditions like hypothyroidism or polycystic ovary syndrome, which also increase predisposition to weight gain. Probably the worst affliction when it comes to difficulty with weight loss is resistance to a hormone called leptin. Leptin, in simple terms, tells your brain you are full, and if you are resistant to it, your brain thinks you are hungry pretty much all the time.

MEDICATION FOR WEIGHT LOSS

The Mayo Clinic (2022) conducted an investigation into weight loss through pharmaceutical drugs obtained by prescriptions from doctors, i.e., drugs that cannot be bought off the shelf. They looked at who should or could be candidates for prescribed weight-loss drugs and concluded the following: If you have not been able to lose weight through diet and exercise and your BMI is greater than 30, you have what would be considered too much body fat, and are classed as obese. This is not always a diagnosis of morbid obesity, but if you do have illnesses classed as comorbidities, then it is safe to say—but unfortunate at the same time—your overall health is at a serious risk.

If you are in a situation as described above, you should definitely see a doctor and request a full medical examination. The doctor will do their assessment and may prescribe medication, say, for high blood pressure. You will need to be informed of the advantages and disadvantages of the medication. Essentially, the disadvantages would be the possible side effects.

In terms of actual weight-loss drugs—i.e., not medication to treat a specific associated condition, but rather medication for the sole purpose of weight loss—there is debate as to how effective they are. A leading study used a weight-loss drug and a placebo in a trial that ran for 12 weeks. It could be argued that the expected results were arrived at. The actual drug did lead to significant weight loss, while the placebo had no effect. Use of weight-loss drugs for 1 year has shown to produce a loss of somewhere between 3% and 12% of body weight. The interesting, but also semi-disappointing finding is that obese individuals who made changes to their lifestyle actually lost less weight than the prescription drug users (Mayo Clinic Staff, 2022).

Some may see these results as positive, and you could say the medication method is best executed with the guidance and advice of a medical professional, but I still strongly feel it is not the way to go. If pharmaceutical drugs are taken for the purposes of treating a genetic weight condition, then I have no issue, but doing so instead of exercising is a cop-out. I understand my view may seem harsh; however, the truth is often harsh but needs to be heard.

The U.S. Food and Drug Administration (FDA) has six weight-loss drugs on its approved list, as follows:

- liraglutide (Saxenda)
- naltrexone/bupropion (Contrave)
- orlistat (Xenical, Alli)
- phentermine/topiramate (Qsymia)
- semaglutide (Wegovy)
- setmelanotide (Imcivree)

I am not going to go into the side effects of each drug individually, but here is a selection from across the board:

- swollen or irritated skin causing red spots and dryness
- patches of darker skin
- nausea
- diarrhea
- belly pain
- unwanted sexual side effects
- depression
- suicidal thoughts

Just by listing some of the side effects, I hope to put off readers from this route to weight loss.

GASTRIC BYPASS SURGERY

In the 1990s and the early 2000s, there was a trend where obese and overweight individuals would seek gastric bypass surgery or gastric sleeve surgery. These methods were popularized by celebrities such as Mariah Carey, Sharon Osborne, and Rosie O'Donnell.

A gastric bypass operation changes the way in which your small intestine and your stomach deal with the food and drink you consume. After the surgery has been completed, your small intestine and your stomach do not process all of the food you ingest. In addition, you tend to feel fuller with less food intake, and thus your body absorbs fewer calories.

Gastric bypass surgery involves two steps. Firstly, staples are used to divide your stomach into two sections. The smaller, walnut-sized section receives the food you eat, and the "feeling fuller faster" result is due to the small size of this section. Next comes the actual bypass, where part of your small intestine is connected to the smaller section of your stomach. The remaining part of the small intestine is bypassed, resulting in the "less calorie absorption" status.

Risks Involved

In 2008 and 2009, gastric bypass surgery in the United States reached a plateau at approximately 113,000 surgeries per annum (Livingstone, 2010). Anastomotic leakage, which is when body fluids leak from where the surgical connection is situated, occurs in about 1.5% to 6% of patients (Gessler et al., 2017) , which means approximately 1,700 to 7,000 people in the US per year experience the related symptoms.

The symptoms are as follows:

- rapid heart rate or sudden drops and rises in heart rate
- fever and stomach pain
- surgical wound drainage

- nausea and vomiting
- left shoulder pain
- low blood pressure
- decreased urine output

The risks of anastomotic leakage increase if you have had previous abdominal surgery. Men are also more at risk, and the heavier you are, the greater the risk becomes.

In addition to the above, bleeding and infections are very likely, and, if not treated, can be life threatening. Other complications include ulcers and pneumonia. The treatments are relatively intricate. Antibiotics administered through an IV line can be used, or a further operation performed. A temporary stent can be placed across the leaking area, and oral intake of food and liquid stopped, to be replaced by a tube directly into your intestine until the leak has healed.

GASTRIC SLEEVE SURGERY

Also called a sleeve gastrectomy, this surgical procedure removes the part of the stomach that usually produces a hormone called ghrelin, which stimulates the appetite. Statistically, people who undergo this surgery are able to lose between 50% and 70% of their excess weight within 24 months of the procedure (Gessler et al., 2017).

Gastrectomies are a measure to alleviate or improve weight-related health problems associated with obesity, i.e., stroke, cancer, heart disease, high blood pressure, high cholesterol, type 2 diabetes, and sleep apnea. Surgeons will usually recommend a gastrectomy only if you have previously tried to lose weight by changing your lifestyle, including exercise. Therefore, you can't expect to have the operation and do nothing thereafter. You will need to eat in a healthy way, and you will have to exercise.

Risks Involved

Like gastric bypass surgery, the gastric sleeve operation poses risks—some long-term and some short-term. These risks include:

- acid reflux
- anesthesia-related risks
- chronic nausea and vomiting
- dilation of the esophagus
- inability to eat certain foods
- infection
- obstruction of the stomach
- dumping syndrome—the combination of a set of symptoms, namely nausea and dizziness, diarrhea, and rapid gastric emptying
- low blood sugar
- malnutrition
- vomiting
- ulcers
- bowel obstruction

- hernias (Woźniewska et al., 2021)

The risks outweigh the rewards by a large margin, and these surgeries are akin to shortcuts. To prevent these risks you should consider returning to the preferred method of eating better and exercising—the healthy way to lose weight!

WEIGHT LOSS AND EXERCISE

Take an event like the Tour de France or track events like the 100 meters. There are trainers, physiotherapists, dieticians, and experts in every aspect of producing athletes who are faster than the next. Weight loss is not necessarily the primary concern in conditioning world-class athletes. However, we now have the knowledge and the means to understand the practical effects of exercise, whether used for weight loss, weight maintenance, or building muscle mass. People in general—professional athletes or otherwise—lose weight more efficiently through eating different foods. Horses for courses. This is where dieticians step in and develop different eating plans for different people. I would just like to make it clear that diet does not mean "a diet" in this instance, but rather what you eat. Essentially, there is no "one size fits all" weight-loss plan.

There is a section in Chapter 7 where I set out the "traditional" exercise types to maintain your ideal weight.

However, getting to your ideal weight is often not achieved through jogging, cycling, or swimming, especially if you are seriously obese. What follows are some exercise suggestions that can be done in the first phase of weight loss. My advice would be to get to a weight where you can walk for 1 kilometer; at this stage you can add the exercise options in Chapter 7 to the ones I am about to explain.

Chair Exercises

One benefit of seated exercises is they put an almost negligible amount of strain on the joints. Another benefit is you can do chair exercises at home. Having been overweight, I understand it can be embarrassing to go to the gym or to exercise in a public place. If you feel the same way, then firstly, you should flip this embarrassment around and make it a positive motivator, after which you can start with some seated exercises.

Choose a comfortable chair that will allow your knees to be positioned at a 90-degree angle. Keep your back straight, with your chin up and your eyes facing forward. You will need to maintain your position and posture for all the following exercises.

Back-and-Forth Slides

Put a paper plate under each foot, slide your left foot forward as far as you can, then bring it back to the 90-

degree starting position. Switch to your right foot and do the same thing. Do 16 reps on each leg and then another 16 with both legs at the same time, moving in alternate directions, as if you were ice-skating. Your goal should be to increase from one set of 16 reps on each leg (plus 16 reps of both legs simultaneously) to two sets, but only when you're ready. These exercises engage your hamstrings and will also get your heart rate up, which is a crucial part of weight loss.

Alternating Toe-Taps

For this exercise, you will need a resistance band. This is basically a big rubber band used during various workouts and can be bought at any sports shop. You will need to wrap the band around your thighs. Then, push your right foot out to the side, tap it down, and return it to the original position. The resistance band creates a pushback, meaning a level of exertion is required. Repeat with the left foot. Complete one set of 16 reps on each side, working up to two sets.

Leg Extensions

From your seated position, lift up your right leg as high as you can before bringing it back down to its original position. Do the same with your left leg, then repeat 20 times. You can look to add ankle weights after a few weeks or a month, when the exercise starts becoming easier—the same goes for increasing the number of sets.

Ball Taps

Usually this exercise is done with a medicine ball, but you can use anything able to withstand a tap with the back of your heel. Place the ball in front of you, lift up your right leg, tap your heel on the medicine ball, and bring it back to its starting position. Either do 16 reps on one leg and then the other, or alternate between legs. Increase the number of sets when you start becoming fitter.

Inner Thigh Squeeze

Place a basketball or similar size object between your knees. Squeeze in as hard as you can, hold for a second, and release. Start with one set of 16 and work your way up.

Resistance Band Lat Pulls

Hold a resistance band above your head and pull your right arm down to your rib cage. Return to your original starting position and do the same with your left arm. One set of 20 reps on each side is advisable at first, to be increased as you start getting fitter.

Seated Lateral Raises

You will need light dumbbells for this exercise, somewhere between 1.5 kg and 2.5 kg. Hold one dumbbell in each hand with your elbows tucked into your waist. Lift each arm straight up in turn, right then left, and repeat 16 times for one set until you get strong enough to increase the number of sets.

Overhead Presses

These are very similar to the seated lateral raises above, except the up-and-down dumbbell movement must be a stretch as high as you can above your head. Either raise each arm one by one, or both arms at the same time. Start with one set of 16 reps and work up to two sets.

Bicep Curls

Use the same weights as the previous two exercises. Tuck your elbows into your sides with your lower arms stretched out at a 90 degree angle, with your palms facing upward. Lift your arm up to your shoulder and then return it to the original position. Twenty reps per arm will do the trick, and you can vary the curls arm by arm or do 20 on one arm followed by 20 on the other, always with the aim of increasing to two sets when you are ready.

Tricep Extensions

You will need the resistance band again for this one. Hold the band out in front of you with your elbows bent and palms face down. Straighten your right arm until it is parallel to the ground, then switch to your left arm and repeat back and forth for 16 reps, again aiming to get up to two sets.

Ab Rotations

This one can be tough, so to start, you are looking at 12 reps. Stretch out your arms parallel to the ground with one of your dumbbells held in both hands. Rotate your torso to the right, as far as you can go, then return to the starting position and do the same rotation to your left—this completes one rep. See if you can get yourself up to two reps.

The Exercise–Weight Loss Research History

In the early 1990s, there was a drive to figure out how much fuel it takes to make a human operate in a highly functional manner. In other words, the mission was to establish how much energy the average human body requires to function at an ongoing optimum level. We get energy from food, but the food has to be metabolized to produce energy. Oxygen helps with metabolizing, but what remains is housed in the liver as fat or glycogen. The latter is a form of carbohydrate. When the liver becomes too full, what cannot be housed is then stored in the body's fat cells. The carbon dioxide we exhale, along with feces and urine, gets rid of waste products. Some people have more efficient systems than others, and our systems operate differently under different conditions.

Early on, the best way to gauge how much energy a person expended was to measure their food and drink intake and track their weight. This would usually be done over a 14-day period. Otherwise, a calorimeter would be used, where a person would be put in a sealed room and have their oxygen inhalation and carbon dioxide exhalation measured. The problem with both methods is that they don't replicate everyday life.

Another approach was to have an individual consume doubly labeled water, which contains oxygen and a harmless isotope called deuterium. After consumption of the water, and over a 7- to 14-day period, the body would excrete oxygen and deuterium in the urine, allowing samples to be collected. The samples would indicate the number of calories burned on a daily basis. This novel method has been used sparingly due to the cost of doubly labeled water, but the net results of these studies have repeatedly indicated that men of average height and typical weight need to burn 2,500 calories per day to maintain a healthy weight. A woman of average height and typical weight has a smaller muscle mass than a man, meaning 2,000 calories per day will facilitate maintenance of a healthy weight (Roberts & Das, 2017).

Lack of Equality in Calories

The three major components of food are proteins, fats, and carbohydrates. You may recall my previous statement that fat actually contains more calories per gram than carbs. This was discovered by Wilber O. Atwater as far back as the 1890s. One gram of fat contains 9 calories, while one gram of protein or carbohydrates contains 4 calories. These numbers are known as the Atwater factors (Roberts & Das, 2017).

Remember, foods and drinks typically are not made up of only one of the components (fat, protein, and carbohydrates). Milk, for instance, contains all three. A study on the topic found that, depending on how nuts are processed, we may have trouble extracting all the calories as stipulated on the product label. For instance, raw almonds eaten whole yield a calorie intake of about a third of the indication on the nutrition label. Taking those nuts and making almond butter, on the other hand, facilitates absorption of all the calories stipulated on the label (Baer & Novotny, 2018).

The whole point of this study was to confirm the hypothesis that not all calories are equal, and it succeeded in doing so. With the confirmation of this inequality, it is easier to understand energy in a human sense.

Energy Expenditure While Resting and While Exercising

Physical activity, contrary to early belief, is only responsible for one-third of energy expenditure. The other two-thirds, called the basal metabolism, represents the energy expended to maintain our body while at rest. As we get older, our rates of metabolism change, and we don't need as many calories to operate as we did when we were younger. Metabolic rate also changes from individual to individual, so the 2,500 calories per day to maintain a healthy weight for men and 2,000 calories for women to do the same are somewhat variable (remember, they are based on the variables of "average" and "typical"). Losing weight also results in your metabolic rate and calorie requirements decreasing because there is "less of you," and, thus, less energy is required. If we take all these possible factors into account, it is relatively safe to conclude that energy expenditure in calories varies in the range of approximately 500 per day.

Hunger in the Brain

From a human evolutionary standpoint, hunger is a message from the brain telling us to eat so we can stay alive. As an advanced civilization, we have easy access to food, as opposed to hunter-gatherer days, when the two main objectives were to find food and not get eaten by predators. Greasy takeaways, chocolate, and fizzy drinks were just not an option. On the one hand, to manage a healthy lifestyle, we need to remove temptation and prevent hunger. A chocolate next to your bed is going to be difficult to resist, but having none in the house removes this temptation. On the hunger front, we need to be eating the *right* foods, which will prolong the periods between the points at which our brains tell us we are hungry or we must eat.

Meals that are higher in fiber and foods that don't spike glucose levels will keep us fuller for longer. Although this is factual, the fundamental problem is food addiction, where individuals will eat even if they are not hungry. This is where willpower or temptation come into focus. Food addiction is considered a mental illness by many, and therapy is highly recommended. If you can work through whatever you are struggling with mentally instead of suppressing it by eating, then you are already removing temptation. Eating, health, and weight loss are person specific, which is fundamentally why diets don't work; furthermore, we need to create health plans based on the individual person, rather than using general health plans in a one size fits all kind of way.

CHAPTER SUMMARY

Clustering is the practice of combining, for our purposes, lifestyle risk factors, the most prevalent of which are smoking, excessive alcohol intake, lack of exercise, and lack of vegetable and fruit intake. The impact of these factors is evidence based, but there are also some untruths regarding weight loss. Not all calories are equal, as we now know, and carbohydrates don't necessarily cause you to become fat. Weight loss directed by supplements is a rarity, and eating fatty foods does not typically make you obese. Fast food is not always fattening, and, to all intents and purposes, diets rarely work. There is no getting around the fact that exercise helps in weight loss. Energy expenditure in addition to calorie losses due to exercise is called the basal metabolism and accounts for approximately two-thirds of energy expenditure. Every single person has experienced the feeling of hunger, and this feeling comes from the brain. However, this does not mean the brain is telling us to eat and drink junk!

We now understand that not everything we hear about weight loss is true, but also that science and research studies are ever-evolving exercises revealing more and more about effective and healthy methods of weight loss. As I mentioned, a lot of the health game is mental, and we can be held back by what we think. Saying things like, "I have a slow metabolism, I'll never lose weight," "I have a body type that is not conducive to weight loss," or "I can't resist the temptation of food" is not going to help. If you truly believe you can't lose weight and you can't get healthy, then you won't—let's dispel some of those beliefs!

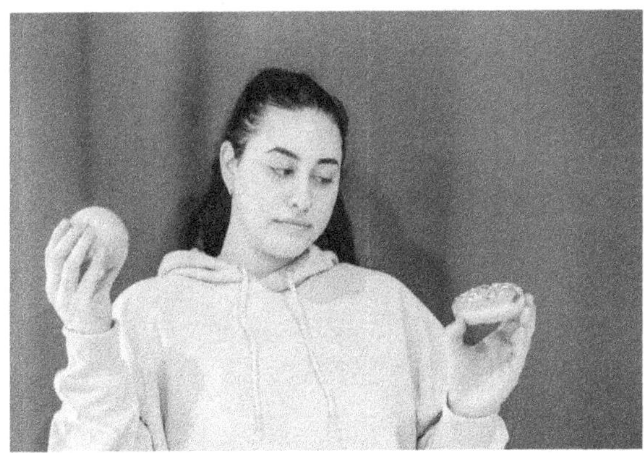

4

STOP BELIEVING YOU CAN'T

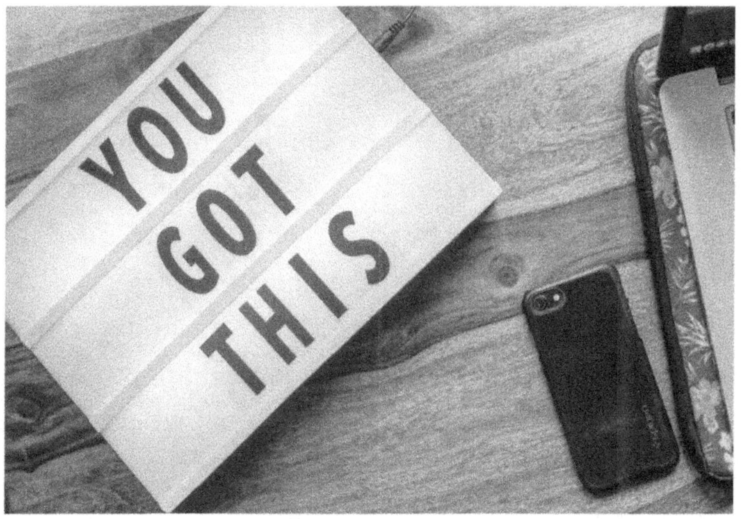

The following quote is not about health or weight loss, but rather about changing the mindset saying you can't do something. It is from Golda Meir, a former teacher and Israeli politician: "Trust yourself. Create the kind of self you will be happy to live with all your life.

Make the most of yourself by fanning the tiny, inner sparks of possibility into flames of achievement" (Haden, 2015).

The part to focus on is the inner spark of possibility. Just a tiny spark of "I can," even if it is smaller than your "I can't," has the potential to become "I did." Wouldn't it be amazing to be able to say you used to believe weight loss and a healthy lifestyle were beyond your realm of possibility, but you overcame this belief and succeeded in spite of it? It definitely would—and it is time to find out how to do so.

UNDERSTANDING METABOLISM

In a rudimentary sense, metabolism is a continuous set of chemical interactions within our cells. The chemicals convert the food we eat into the energy required to operate the machine that is the human body. Our metabolic rate changes at different times of the day and is influenced by more factors than you might think. Within the auspices of metabolism, there are two interactive systems at work.

Catabolism

This term originates in the ancient Greek language (which developed into New Latin), and translates roughly as "downward." This makes sense, as catabolism is the breaking down of food components. Catabolism has been referred to as "destructive metabolism" because it is the tearing apart of proteins, carbohydrates, and fats to produce cellular activity through energy. Along with the good comes the bad, meaning catabolism also produces the waste products released from our bodies in the form of sweat, urine, feces, and the carbon dioxide we expel when breathing out.

Anabolism

The growth of new cells, the storage of energy, and the maintenance of body tissues are all taken care of by anabolism. Anabolic steroids, of which I am certain you have heard, are supplements that advance anabolism; this is why they (or most of them) are on the banned substance list when it comes to professional sports. This was not always the case, especially when they first hit the market and were largely experimentative.

Catabolism and Anabolism Working Together

Catabolism and anabolism are somewhat of a team, instructed by the body's nervous system and hormonal system. Every human body has a metabolic rate, which differs from person to person and changes throughout the day, depending on several factors. Metabolism is complex, so let's break it down into three factors and deconstruct them to create clarity.

Basal Metabolic Rate

I touched on this briefly, but as a reminder, your BMR describes the kilojoules your body burns when it is at rest. BMR is the amount of energy required for your body to maintain itself. BMR is linked to your lean mass, which, in simple terms, is the weight of everything excluding fat—i.e., muscle, body water, bones, skin, and organs. Anything that results in a reduction of lean mass is directly proportional to the reduction of BMR. This is why you always want to maintain muscle mass when you are trying to lose weight. BMR represents 50% to 80% of total energy use, and you want to be as high as possible on this spectrum. The average man has a BMR of approximately 7,100 kilojoules per day, while the average woman sits at around 5,900 kilojoules per day.

Energy Used During Exercise and Physical Activity

Movement and physical activity also call on kilojoules and fuel the muscles with energy during strenuous exercise. The rate of energy expenditure is likely to rise by 50 times when your muscles are engaged in exercise or other physical activity. The latter might include carrying heavy tiles for work, as an arbitrary example. Unlike BMR, you have control of energy expenditure through exercise and physical activity, which is why you have the power to exploit control over your weight loss and health improvement endeavors.

The Thermic Effect

This is dead simple—it is the energy used to eat, digest, and metabolize food. Yes, chewing requires energy, and so does the digestion and metabolization of what you chew (and swallow). Logically, eating spikes your metabolism. The peak is reached approximately 2.5 to 3 hours later. The spike has a large range, starting at about 2% and potentially reaching 30% depending on the food type and meal size. In line with thermic (meaning "thermal," i.e., heat), spicy foods have a relatively high thermic effect.

INCREASING SLOW METABOLISM

First off, starving yourself is a terrible way to lose weight. You will, in fact, lose more muscle, become weaker, and not have much of a good time. Not eating for extended periods does not promote sustainability, and, when you return to eating, there is a strong chance you will eat even more than you did before your fast. There is no absolute formula, and fitness experts and dietitians disagree on certain aspects. One aspect where there seems to be more agreement, though, is the six-meal-a-day method. This makes sense from the point of view that the act of eating, digesting, and metabolizing, as examined in the thermic effect section, increases your metabolism. The six-meal theory states that, by eating this way, your metabolism is being increased six times a day. What you are eating is also important. Six pizzas a day ain't going to do any good, so you need to choose fruit, vegetables, healthy grains, and lean protein. We all know what fruits and vegetables are, but grains maybe not so much. Healthy grains include barley, oats, quinoa, wild rice, rye, whole wheat, and maize, among many others. This is not saying you can never eat a burger, a burrito, or a slice of chocolate cake—of course you can, but *in moderation.*

Smaller Factors That Affect Metabolism

Genes do have an effect on metabolism, and larger people usually need more calories because they have more muscle mass. Gender also plays a role, and men generally have more muscle mass than women.

Sleep helps regulate your glucose levels, so lack of sleep can lead to a lack of energy. It is very difficult to go to sleep at the same time every night and wake up at the same time every morning. Life gets in the way—sometimes we have to work late, some nights we may play indoor sports, and sometimes we are exhausted emotionally and want to go to bed early. Another part of life frowned upon by sleep experts is TV, computers, and phones before bed. You should put them away at least an hour before bedtime and also sleep in a dark room.

FASTING—THE GOOD(-ISH) KIND

When I talked about not eating for long periods earlier, I meant starving yourself for several days with the goal of immediate weight loss. In this section, I am talking about intermittent fasting, usually for periods of 8 hours, although time period recommendations do differ. The reason this works for weight loss is that the body starts to burn fat after it has burned energy, and allowing 8 hours for it to burn energy will inevitably allow your body to move onto fat burning. A practical problem is overcompensation, and people who experience food addiction will identify with this. If something triggers your overeating and it happens during a part of the fasting period, there is a significant chance you will break the fast, but to the point where you end up eating more than you would on an ordinary day. Food addiction means consuming comfort foods, and on days when your mental state triggers the need for food, it is so difficult to maintain willpower.

Back to the good type of fasting—intermittent. In a study into calorie restriction, the three most popular types of intermittent fasting were found to be alternate-day fasting, all-day fasting, and time-restricted feeding:

- Alternate-day fasting involves alternating between days of no food restriction at all, and days where you eat one meal that provides about 25% of your daily calorie needs. As an example, Mondays, Wednesdays, and Fridays would be the "fasting" days, while Tuesdays, Thursdays, Saturdays, and Sundays would be the "alternate days," when there are no food consumption restrictions at all.

- All-day fasting refers to 2 days per week (or 3 days in extreme cases) of complete fasting, or consuming up to 25% of daily calorie needs, with no food restriction on the other 4 or 5 days. For example, the 5:2 diet (2 days of fasting, 5 days unrestricted) approach advocates no food restriction on 5 days of the week, cycled with a 400–500-calorie diet on the other 2 days of the week.

- Time-restricted feeding means following a meal plan each day with a designated time frame for fasting. As an example, meals are eaten between 8 am and 3 pm, with fasting from after the 3 pm meal until the 8 am meal the next morning (Liu et al., 2022).

At the risk of repeating myself, these methods are only effective if kept up indefinitely, and, as you will hear over and over, a balanced diet combined with a comprehensive exercise plan is the best way to lose weight, keep it off, and remain healthy. Yes, intermittent fasting does work, but only among a small set of the population. It is unclear whether intermittent fasting is superior to other weight-loss methods in regards to the amount of weight loss, the biological changes, the compliance rates, and decreased appetite.

If an exercise regime is started in conjunction with the intermittent fasting, weight loss can be rapid, but very unhealthy and energy sapping.

LOSING WEIGHT TOO FAST

When we think of losing weight we generally think of losing fat, but very rapid weight loss can include loss of muscle too, which is the opposite of what our weight loss intentions are—or, at least, should be. We are aware a low-calorie diet will bring on fast weight loss, and a study into losing weight too fast produced some interesting results.

A low-calorie diet was designed by researchers, who put 25 people on an eating plan of 500 calories per day for 5 weeks. A second diet was developed, including a meal plan of 1,250 calories per day for 12 weeks, and was prescribed to 22 people. Both groups lost weight, but the people who followed the 500-calorie intake plan lost over six times as much muscle as those on the 1,250-calorie intake plan. Other than the loss of muscle associated with quick weight loss, it is possible for the body to have other adverse responses. Generally, the immune system will be down, and, combined with energy loss, dehydration, constipation, muscle cramping, and headaches, there can also be a mental health impact (Vink et al., 2016).

To sum it up in one short sentence: Rapid weight loss has too many health dangers and disadvantages to hold any positive recommendations.

HEALTHY EATING ON AN ONGOING BASIS

We know cutting down on food intake will help you lose weight—this is just logic. But, as we also know, exercise must come into it too. The ideal situation is for you to get into the chair exercise routines as above, with the aim of getting to the upright exercises, which we will look at in Chapter 7.

One approach you could take to healthy eating is to largely reduce your volume of food consumption; however, if you usually eat two chocolate bars a day and you reduce it to one chocolate bar per day, that is still too much chocolate. The better bet is to change your diet to something healthy and filling, so you are not dreaming of junk food for half the day. Below are some simple suggestions, which I call a 7-day meal plan, which you can mix and match, improvise, and get creative.

The 7-Day Meal Plan

There are plenty of meal plans out there, and 7-day plans are the most common. Of course, the plan is not just for the first 7 days, but is intended to be repeated as a routine. You do still want to enjoy eating, and in this regard, you do not have to stick to the recommended portions in a militant way. What follows are guidelines divided into five categories: namely, breakfast, morning snack, lunch, afternoon snack, and dinner.

Breakfast

Traditionally, breakfast is referred to as the most important meal of the day. This is a matter of opinion. Nonetheless, here are some good breakfast options:

- Avocado and egg on toast (one to two slices). Rye or whole wheat are the generally recommended types of bread. Carbohydrate-heavy breads like sourdough should be avoided.
- One bowl of bran cereal and blueberries (approximately half a cup of blueberries). Skim milk is advised, but you can also go with low fat instead of full cream, which you should avoid.
- Plain Greek yogurt, spiced up with two teaspoons of honey, a generous sprinkling of almonds, and half a cup of blueberries.
- One cup of rolled oats cooked in a cup of milk (skim or low fat) mixed with a cup of raspberries.

You can mix up the above four meals over the 7 days, or, if you prefer some over others, then just focus on those ones.

Mid-Morning Snack

You should aim to have your morning snack at around 10.30 a.m., but don't be too stringent. Here are some suggested options:

- One cup of blueberries or a cup of blueberries and raspberries mixed.
- One to two medium-sized apples.
- One banana, grapefruit, or pear—whichever you prefer.
- One medium bell pepper, sliced, with three tablespoons of hummus.

Just like with breakfast, you can mix it up with the fruit, depending on which ones you prefer.

Lunch

Lunch should be about 2 hours after your mid-morning snack and could consist of one of the following:

- Black bean nacho soup.
- Large spinach and strawberry salad. You can add tomato, lettuce, parmesan cheese, tuna, and a little bit of salt.
- Tuna salad with white beans and dill.
- Two slices of whole-wheat bread with avocado.

You can mix and match, perhaps adding egg to the avocado bread or replacing the avocado with egg.

Mid-Afternoon Snack

Aim to eat your afternoon snack at around 3.30 p.m. Here are your options:

- One to two medium apples.
- One cup of blueberries.
- One cup of strawberries.
- One cup of blueberries.
- One to two medium oranges.

Just like the previous meals, give preference to the foods you enjoy more, and feel free to eat berry mixes if you choose.

Dinner

The last meal of the day is a bit more complex and also takes a bit of preparation time. I am not going to give you any recipes, but after the chapter summary I will list some reputable websites offering easy recipes. Your other option is to get a cookery book and pick out meals that are the same or similar to the following:

- Salmon with green peppercorn sauce or similar sauce, served with one cup of steamed vegetables and a large baked potato (don't go crazy with the salt and butter, but allow yourself a small indulgence).

- Shrimp, pesto, and quinoa bowl.
- Curried soup—preferably white meat and sweet potato, accompanied by a slice of whole-wheat bread.
- Brown rice and couscous salad. Add some steamed broccoli for a fresh flavor.
- Cauliflower and boiled chicken with mushroom sauce.

You can mix and match those five options or choose three that you particularly like, then repeat them. Be explorative and look for other meals if you like… and yes, one or two chocolate bars per week is fine—in moderation.

METABOLIC DISORDERS

In the context of the world population, the number of people with metabolic disorders is small, but they are out there, and it is unfortunate they exist. Metabolic disorders are almost always inherited genetically, and for the most part are not completely curable. In some cases metabolic diseases can be managed, resulting in a decent quality of life, but for the most part they do cause unpleasantness.

Gaucher Disease

This is a very unpleasant disorder that is responsible for stomach aches, bloating, enlarged organs, anemia, bruising, and excessive bleeding. There are several types of Gaucher disease, but only one type is treatable through medication and enzyme-replacement therapy. Eating well and exercising when you can are recommended, but the latter is difficult to achieve when experiencing the symptoms.

Hemochromatosis

Iron retention and storage are associated with hemochromatosis, which results in pancreas, liver, and heart damage. It is not preventable, but if it is diagnosed at an early stage, it can be treated. Unfortunately, the disease is incurable, but blood removal to reduce iron retention can reverse organ damage or at least slow it down.

Maple Syrup Urine Disease

Foods that contain protein also contain amino acids, which cannot be broken down. As a result, the amino acids become toxic as they start to build up. The disease can be life threatening if not diagnosed very shortly after birth, although very specific protein-absent eating plans can lessen the severity of the symptoms. Severely depleted energy, along with vomiting and poor intellectual development, are the major symptoms, and without medical management, premature death is common.

Mitochondrial Disease

This metabolic disease is more frequently diagnosed than you might suspect, with 1 in every 5,000 people inheriting it genetically. There are a whole host of symptoms, including poor muscle growth, migraines, strokes, heart disease, breathing problems, and dementia. Treatment differs depending on the symptoms displayed, but exercise is encouraged. Vitamin intake can also assist in reducing physical symptoms. However, neurological or mental-health ramifications, dementia being the main one, cannot be treated.

Tay-Sachs Disease

Also a genetic disorder, this is caused by receiving a defective *HEXA* gene (known scientifically as hexosaminidase subunit alpha) from each parent. The disease severely inhibits physical development and motor skills. Genetic testing prior to birth is the only manner in which to detect Tay-Sachs disease. There are a number of variations of the disease, but either way affected children seldom lead long lives.

Wilson's Disease

Wilson's disease is extremely rare and predominantly affects the eyes, brain, and liver. It is characterized by an excess of copper in the body. Symptoms include rings around the eyes, tremors, and abdominal pains via the liver and other internal organs, in addition to mental-health problems, such as anxiety and depression. Treatment involves copper-reducing medication, and although the disease can be partially managed, it can never be cured.

METABOLIC SYNDROME

Heart disease, type 2 diabetes, and strokes can be the end result of cases of metabolic syndrome, which is characterized by several conditions experienced simultaneously: high blood pressure, high blood sugar, abnormal levels of cholesterol, and excess body weight. If you have only one of these conditions, you are still at risk of developing others. One in every three Americans above the age of 18 years is estimated to have metabolic syndrome.

Insulin resistance is a disease linked to metabolic syndrome. What we eat is broken down into sugar. Insulin assists the sugar in making its way into your cells. This is the process. However, insulin-resistant individuals often experience high blood sugar levels after taking insulin to get the sugar into the cells. Insulin rescue can become type 2 diabetes if action is not taken to control your weight and health.

High blood pressure and cholesterol assist in creating plaque, which clogs the arteries. As we discussed previously, this results in hardened and narrowed arteries and can lead to a stroke or a heart attack.

Preventive measures would be jogging, swimming, or engaging in some form of exercise. Between 30- and 45-minute sessions are recommended, and if you can do this five times a week, you will notice a difference. Try to cut out salt or severely reduce your intake. Increase your consumption of fruits and vegetables, as usual, and, finally, limit your fat consumption. The obvious ones are to stop smoking and either cut alcohol out completely, or reduce it significantly.

WEIGHT CYCLING

Otherwise referred to as "yo-yo dieting," weight cycling is up-and-down weight fluctuations, as in gaining and losing weight as a result of starting and stopping different diets. Scientific studies have found a good predictor of future serious illness and death is to look at the dynamics of weight cycling in individuals. Research has also shown weight stability to be the optimum trajectory, so to speak (Lissner & Heitmann, 2013). Using the term "trajectory" is a bit of an anomaly, as this term is usually interpreted as big ups and downs. This isn't incorrect, but very small variations in weight could be said to be an undulating trajectory.

As I am sure you will have noticed, people who are always trying out different fad diets never manage to lose weight. The obvious conclusion is weight cycling has no benefits. Perhaps the exception would be jockeys and boxers who need to control their weight, and sometimes have to use different diets to do so. Don't forget in these sports the level of professionalism and science means yo-yo-ing would be done in the healthiest possible manner; I still do not advise it, though.

BELIEVING IN YOURSELF

Having self-belief and the determination to get healthy and lose weight plays a huge part in the process. It is called a lifestyle change because if you do it properly, you will quite literally become the opposite of your current self, lifestyle-wise. A lot of people say they will do something, such as learning an instrument or playing a new sport, but never actually end up doing it. You need to find your own motivation and not end up in the "say they will" group. Motivation is an ongoing, everyday commitment; it may wane from time to time, but, as resilient human beings, we have the power to re-harness our motivation when it slips.

It may help with motivation if you make daily assertions about your health and the ways to improve it, recognizing a healthy lifestyle is the sum total of a bunch of good habits. You will hear people say if you overeat today then you must cut down the next day. This is absolutely correct —nobody can maintain an eating plan where they never slip up and have a slice of cake at a party, for example. Don't judge yourself when it happens, but tell yourself the next day you will cut something out or eat a smaller dinner. When you get into the swing of things with your exercise routine, and you just have one day where work has gotten you down and exercise is the last thing you want to do, then walk for 5 minutes instead of 30 minutes. Do *something* so you can say you have achieved something. Don't just abandon things—do a little bit rather than doing nothing.

A support network and people who can hold you account-able will help increase and maintain your motivation. Involve your friends and report back to them on your good (and bad) lifestyle choices. Back to the subject of exercise: If you join an exercise class or a walking club, then there are people you will let down if you don't attend. Such is motivation in itself.

Then there is the old trick of putting a photograph of your current self on the fridge, alongside a picture of the way you would like to look. An amazing motivator is when you start to visibly notice your weight is declining and you can feel yourself getting fitter. Hold onto those feelings and, when your motivation is low, remind your-self of how well you are doing.

Chronicle your journey in a diary, read inspirational stories of others who have turned unhealthy lifestyles around, listen to podcasts on exercise and good eating, and talk to people about your intended health transformation. Whatever works for you in terms of motivation—do it!

CHAPTER SUMMARY

Mindset is vital—you really have to want to get healthy. It is easy to say you will be healthy or you will "start exercising from Monday." But, until you have the correct mindset and the accompanying willpower, you will struggle to succeed. Understanding metabolism is a step in the right direction, especially the way in which catabolism and anabolism work together. You already know about the BMR and the energy used during physical activities, but also keep in mind the thermic effect—the energy used to eat, digest, and metabolize food.

Intermittent fasting *can* work, but it has to be maintained, and, in a global sense, the evidence does not conclude whether intermittent fasting works. Then there are the metabolic disorders, inherited genetically, which I am not going to go into in this summary—you can refer back to them if need be. Metabolic syndrome brings with it a number of complications due to its nature—several conditions experienced simultaneously. Heart disease, type 2 diabetes, and strokes are common end results of metabolic syndrome. Weight cycling, or yo-yo dieting, is not going to help much. As I said earlier in the chapter, people who are always trying different diets don't lose weight.

Well, you know all about metabolism now, and I am confident you have learned a lot. There were definitely a few wake-up calls in this chapter, and I hope they can become your motivation to push aside "diets." It is sad that some people have diseases like mitochondrial disease and Gaucher diseases. We should do as much as we can to help those people by being examples to them and inspiring them to live the new healthy life you are living.

Now, it is time to uncover some of the mystery surrounding diets. As promised, here is a list of some of the most reputable recipe websites, compiled in March 2023:

- allrecipes.com
- bbcgoodfood.com
- chefkoch.de
- cookpad.com
- foodnetwork.com
- kurashiru.com
- marmiton.org
- tasteofhome.com

Below are five of the top best-selling cooking books to consider buying:

- *10-Minute Recipes: Fast Food, Clean Ingredients, Natural Health,* by Liana Werner-Gray
- *The Doctor's Kitchen: Supercharge Your Health with 100 Delicious Everyday Recipes,* by Dr. Rupy Aujla
- *The Whole30 Fast and Easy Cookbook: 150 Simply Delicious Everyday Recipes for Your Whole30,* by Melissa Hartwig
- *The World's Fittest Book,* by Ross Edgely
- *The How Not to Die Cookbook: Over 100 Recipes to Help Prevent and Reverse Disease,* by Dr. Michael Greger

My Weight Loss Journey

"The first wealth is health."

— RALPH WALDO EMERSON

Total Health Weight Loss Redefined is a book that takes a fresh and comprehensive approach to losing weight and achieving sustainable results.

It goes beyond the usual advice of diet and exercise, delving into the realms of psychology, nutrition science, and lifestyle modification to create a well-rounded and effective weight loss journey.

I present a unique perspective on weight loss that challenges old ideas and empowers individuals to take control of their health and happiness. Through easy-to-understand explanations, practical tips, and inspiring real-life stories,

Total Health Weight Loss Redefined equips readers with the tools they need to break free from unhealthy habits and create lasting change.

To make that change happen, I have a question for you...

Would you help someone you've never met, even if you never got credit for it?

Who is this person you ask? They are like you. Or, at least, like you used to be. Less experienced, wanting to make a difference, and needing help, but not sure where to look.

Our mission is to make Total Health Weight Loss Redefined accessible to everyone. Everything we do stems from that mission. And, the only way for us to accomplish that mission is by reaching everyone.

This is where you come in. Most people do, in fact, judge a book by its cover (and its reviews). So, here's my ask on behalf of a struggling man or woman failing with weight loss you've never met:

Please help that man or woman by leaving this book a review.

Your gift costs no money and less than 60 seconds to make real, but can change a fellow man or woman's life forever. Your review could help…

To get that 'feel good' feeling and help this person for real, all you have to do is...and it takes less than 60 seconds...leave a review.

5

THE MYSTERIES OF DIETS

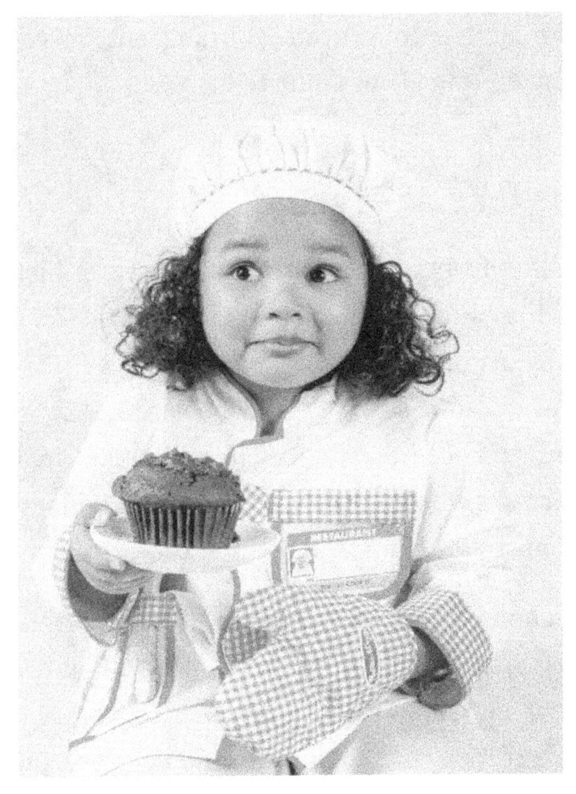

Diets certainly have a colorful history. We know fundamentally they do not work, and I would like to reiterate that eating in moderation is not "dieting" or "following a diet." Diet, as in an eating plan or strategy, carries with it the reputation that you may lose weight, but you won't keep up the diet. We need to maintain a healthy diet and accompany it with exercise.

I keep telling you diets don't work; however, I have been pretty vague until now. I hope you have been looking forward to this section because it is imperative to know all the ins and outs and the different reasons they don't work. My aim is to educate you and ensure you 100% realize fad dieting is not going to help you.

THE HISTORY OF DIETING

I am willing to bet you didn't know the first historically identified book on dieting was published in 1558. It was written by an Italian national named Luigi Cornaro. His book was called *The Art of Living Long*, and it is still in print today. The diet is very simple, which makes one wonder how a whole book was written: 12 ounces of food and 14 ounces of wine per day—that's it.

It took another 172 years for the next diet book to be published. The title was *The Natural Method of Curing the Diseases of the Body*, and it was written by Dr. George Cheyne, a British physician. Milk and vegetables were the doctor's staples, and they did help him lose weight, but as you could guess, when he returned to normal eating all the weight—and more—returned.

The first diet influencer is said to be Lord Byron, arguably one of the world's greatest poets. During the Victorian era, Byron was considered a man of beauty. His diet plan included starving himself for a period, followed by binge eating, followed by wearing several layers of warm clothing to sweat out what he had consumed. What a terrible idea! But, to give him some credit, much less was known about health in the 18th and 19th centuries than today.

As time progressed, the low-carb diet was popularized in 1825 and is the basis for the keto, paleo, and Atkins diets, which are still used today. One could thus say some diets have not changed for centuries... and what does this tell us? I will leave the answer up to you.

DOES DIETING MAKE YOU FAT?

This question has been asked many times over, and has been discussed at great length. A fascinating and informative study in 2011 attempted to answer the question. One of the interesting parts of the study was that 4,129 individual twins participated. Of course, not every individual was a "dieter"; nevertheless, they still contributed to the study in terms of data collected about balanced diets and good health. The objective of the study was to look into whether gaining or losing weight is more closely related to genetics.

Interestingly, 90% of the twins were Finnish and were born between 1975 and 1979. You could argue that the study should have probed nationality or upbringing based on area as a factor. However, the research was focused on genetic weight loss only. As you can imagine, the study wasn't particularly easy to carry out, but researchers recorded height and weight when the sets of twins were 16, 17, and 18 years old. They were then measured again at 25 years of age, including what they referred to as intentional weight loss (IWL). The IWL ceiling was 5 kg or more, and the idea was to measure the history of IWL from age 16 to age 25. There were conclusions on several areas of weight loss and weight gain, but the one pertinent for our purposes was the following: Frequent IWL reflects susceptibility to weight gain, rendering dieters more prone to future weight gain (Pietiläinen et al, 2012).

Several studies over the years have garnered similar results, and an article published on Healthline entitled *Do 'Diets' Really Just Make You Fatter?* gives readers an accurate perspective in answering the question. It looked at the monetization side of the weight-loss industry and, using data from various studies, it put forward the fact that the American and European weight-loss markets had created over $150 billion in profits in 2015. The article made a prediction that the $150 billion figure would grow to $256 billion by 2022 (Spritzler, 2020).

A 2014 study found the average financial cost of losing 11 pounds (5 kg) ranged from $755 for the WeightWatchers program to $2,730 for the medication route (Finkelstein & Kruger, 2014). It wouldn't be naive to assume most of the weight lost is gained again, and the methods used by WeightWatchers don't work on a long-term basis.

Logically, if every person completed a diet, lost the weight desired, and kept it off, the above numbers and figures would look vastly different. Going back to Spritzler's article, she draws a similar conclusion and suggests spending money chasing weight loss is "without long term success."

Three quoted studies which delved into diet success rates produced the following results:

- After 3 years from the date of completing a weight-loss program, only 12% of participants had kept off at least 75% of the weight they had lost, while 40% had gained back more weight than they had originally lost (Grodstein et al., 1996).
- Five years after a group of women lost weight during a 6-month controlled weight-loss program, they weighed 7.9 pounds (3.6 kg) more than their starting weight on average (Foster et al., 1996).
- In many cases, weight regain may be higher than reported because follow-up rates are very low, and weight is often self-reported by phone or mail (Mann et al., 2007).

The results of these studies are indicative of the fact diets do not work—and the Mann study paints the picture as even worse, given follow-up rates and self-reporting. We can never say diets absolutely do not work in the long term, but we can say, in the context of the results of various studies, it is very rare to see effective weight-loss working for long-term periods. So, what should we do to lose weight, based on these statistics? I will tell you—look at alternatives that actually work.

Healthy Choices

I can sum it up by telling you to reduce your calorie intake and to eat foods that sustain you for longer, but there is much more to it. Every day we are bombarded with adverts for junk food, fizzy drinks, alcohol, and other glorified but unhealthy choices. Manufacturers don't care about our health; they care about our money. I would venture to say every single reader has seen a billboard advertising a chocolate bar, a fried-chicken meal, or a fat-soaked burrito, and made a left turn to the nearest outlet. We do have the power to choose, and I would advise, when a craving hits or you start considering eating a really unhealthy meal, you stop to consider the options and their ramifications. Here is an example of an internal conversation you can use to help you make a good health choice:

Yes, I really want to have a big KFC meal. How will I feel afterward? Probably guilty, and when this feeling hits it will be too late. So, will the whole experience be a good one? No, there will be a few minutes of pleasure while eating, followed by the awful feeling of guilt. What are my other choices? A chicken salad from the Pioneer Chicken Stand around the corner.

As time goes by and you have more internal conversations like this, which lead to the healthier choice, good habits will start forming. As soon as you feel better in yourself, you will want to maintain the feeling, which comes from good eating and exercising.

Mindful Eating

Mindfulness is the concept of being completely present and absorbed in a moment or while doing something. When applied to eating, you can focus on the aromas, savor every bite, and identify the different flavors. Eat slowly and deeply enjoy the experience; plus, the more slowly you eat, the fuller you get. We can also apply this to meal preparation—set the scene in a clean kitchen with some music playing, and take your time as you chop, slice, boil, garnish, and bake.

Exercise

You don't even have to do a whole lot of exercise. Research suggests at least 30 minutes of daily physical activity is particularly beneficial for weight maintenance (Nakata et al., 2014). Finding 30 minutes out of 24 hours should not be difficult. Perhaps motivation is a bigger factor than time, but when you have been at it for 10 days, or maybe 2 weeks, you will start to love how you feel! Chapter 7 sets out some different exercise options. Not everyone enjoys exercise, but it is necessary, and can become enjoyable depending on the exercise you choose and your mindset toward it.

FAD DIETS

I have mentioned fad diets a few times, but what exactly are they? A fad in general is short lived—a craze, if you like. The problem with these fad diets is that your body will be robbed of the nutrients needed to stay healthy. So, even though you might lose weight, the negative health impacts will likely be profound. Often, research on a particular diet is lacking, but you have to remember the people and companies who promote fad diets are really just looking to make money.

Signs of a fad diet that is unlikely to produce the results it professes to do are claims the weight loss can be immediate, or relatively so. If it sounds too good to be true, there is a huge chance it really is. Often when marketing fad diets, companies that sell weight-loss products or monetize those products in some way will refer to studies that actually don't exist, or will quote legitimate studies but manipulate the way in which the conclusions are framed.

You may also notice weight-loss product companies making recommendations to sell a book or books related to their product. This is also a sign of a fad diet, possibly combined with some clever, but dishonest, marketing. It is a bit of a double-edged sword, because some recommendations as a selling technique are credible—it is up to you as the consumer to make the distinction, though.

If you are unsure, you can look for peer-reviewed studies into the diet or product (peer review is basically when a professional in the same field examines a study and gives critical analysis and approval). Some quoted studies will not differentiate between, for example, men and women, but just make general claims. As you will have picked up from the studies referred to previously, a lot of different factors come into the research. Sometimes, fad-diet promoters will make claims that one of the five food groups (fruits, vegetables, grains, protein foods, and dairy) is not good for you and that they should be removed from your eating plan. Finally, testimonials, such as "I lost 20 pounds in only 14 days without exercising," should be treated with skepticism.

Fad diets are, for all intents and purposes, crash diets. I must reiterate that I strongly disagree with them. However, it would be remiss of me not to tell you how they *can* work. To repeat myself again, fad and/or crash diets are unhealthy. I want my position on this to be clear. In any event, if you fast for 48 hours, say from dinner on Sunday night until dinner on Tuesday night, followed by a series of 24-hour fasts between Wednesday and Saturday, you will lose weight. In order to keep it off, you would have to introduce an intense exercise regime at the same time, because if you did the "diet" for 2 weeks, then stopped and went back to eating junk food, the weight gain would be almost as fast as the loss. The idea should be to get to a weight below your ideal, then maintain the intense exercising while slowly returning to a balanced (and healthy) diet.

MOST UNBELIEVABLE FAD DIETS

Some fads are crazier than others, but over time there have been some really ridiculous fad diets, all of which are definitely on the "never try these" list. We still need to have a look at them, partially for entertainment value, but mostly to put you off trying them.

The Cigarette Diet

Lucky Strike cigarettes in the 1920s had an ad campaign with the slogan, "Reach for a Lucky Instead of a Sweet." It worked as a marketing ploy but didn't do much for lung and chest health—although in this era doctors were recommending cigarette smoking, so we can't be too critical of those who subscribed to this diet. There is a school of thought that nicotine suppresses your appetite, but there is another school of thought suggesting smoking is just a distraction from food. Whatever the case, smoking has only negative consequences, and I am not even going to get on to vaping. Stay away!

The Sleeping Beauty Diet

There isn't much to say about this one—sleep as much as you can, and you will shed weight. It is unclear if the thinking was you can't eat while you are asleep, and therefore you won't put on any weight, or if the process of sleeping itself was seen as a kilo cutter. Sleeping away your life is not the most productive way to function, and is unlikely to contribute to a healthier lifestyle. It is quite unbelievable that certain people considered this a viable method, but thank goodness we are all different.

The Master Cleanse Diet

This diet also eliminates food and focuses on consuming a drink made up of maple syrup, lemon juice, water, and cayenne pepper. The latter ingredient contains capsaicin, which was said to be a fat-burning component. It gets more bizarre, though—the diet starts with a laxative salt water cleanse, followed by 12 glasses of the four-ingredient drink. You will lose weight, but the reason for this will be the lack of eating, so the weight won't stay off for long after regular eating is resumed.

The Baby Food Diet

This crazy diet recommends several jars of baby food for breakfast and lunch, followed by a normal meal at dinner. This diet limits intake of the protein and nutrients required by an adult body and also works off the premise of starving yourself to shed the kilos. And we all know what happens when regular eating is picked up again…

The Cabbage Soup Diet

This classic is a 7-day plan that involves eating only cabbages and cabbage soup. Some people add in other vegetables, but either way, I don't need to tell you what happens from day 8 onward, and rapidly so.

The Tapeworm Diet

This one is definitely disgusting! You eat tapeworm eggs, which hatch in your gastrointestinal tract. These newly hatched tapeworms are said to eat the food you ingest as it passes through your gastrointestinal tract, thus causing you to lose weight. It is almost impossible to believe people do this, but people get desperate and will try anything. Please don't try this… ever!

BETTER OPTIONS

Before we look at the options, I would like to tell you the story of Lindsey Bone and a ridiculous diet, if one can call it that. Lindsey was a British student who was found dead by friends with whom she shared a residence. Lindsey was 20 years old at the time and had been on an extreme plan to lose weight before an upcoming holiday. She engaged in fasting for significant periods, combined with taking apple cider vinegar supplements in tablet form. It could be said that Lindsey starved herself to death, and although the coroner's report was not officially released, the cause of death was very obvious. Lindsey's story should come as a shock and also act as a warning—going to such extremes is exceptionally dangerous to your health.

It is much more responsible and advisable to make small changes at first. Cutting down on sugar intake is an excellent start. In fact, if you can get into the habit of minimizing sugar consumption, you will adjust quickly, and what would have formerly been a normal amount of sugar will become an excessive amount as far as your taste buds are concerned. Also, don't demonize foods. You can still eat them, but cut down on them rather than carry on hating yourself for indulging in excess. A medium pizza, as opposed to a large one, is a good "cut down." There are days on which you will eat more than others, and you shouldn't be too judgmental of yourself as long as you cut down the next day to bring in the balance—I strongly believe in this. Don't be resistant to seeing a dietitian. They are experts and can help you with an eating plan (not a diet) that fits *you* best. Exercise, too—you know that! But I will mention it again anyway!

CHAPTER SUMMARY

I think it is safe to say, thanks to proper research and study, you should be convinced diets do not work. The science is irrefutable, and the research does not lie. Years of studies and weight-related monitoring, as well as the monetization of the diet industry to the extent that it has been monetized, are indicators pointing to only one thing. The diet industry in the United States and Europe is worth over $150 billion annually—and if all the products, weight-loss clubs, supplements, and diets really worked, the amount would be significantly lower.

The choice is yours, and when making decisions about what to eat, you need to get an internal dialogue going, where you convince yourself the healthy choice is the correct choice. Mindful eating, which is basically focusing deeply on what you are eating, will prolong and ignite the enjoyment provided by every healthy meal. Adding exercise to your routine is another great choice, which will be vindicated by the rewards of looking and feeling healthy.

Remember to look out for the signs of a fad diet, like big claims and testimonials, or advice requiring you to buy expensive products.

By this point I sincerely hope you are strongly against fad diets, having gained all this knowledge on the subject, and I also hope you can see how the overall health picture is the most important one. Now, we are going to look at the secrets to overall health in the next chapter.

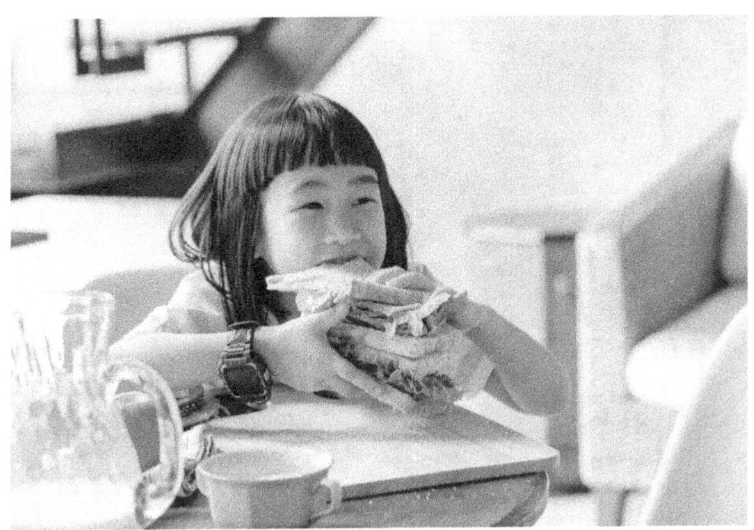

6

SECRETS TO OVERALL HEALTH

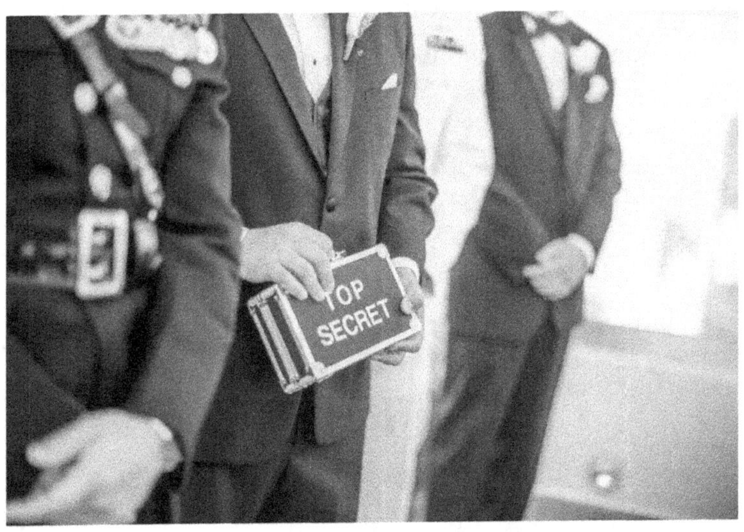

Most of us want to live a relatively long life, but the proviso would be that we only want to live as long as we are healthy. Unfortunately, life-threatening diseases do not discriminate. Young people get cancer, die of heart attacks, or find themselves confined to wheelchairs. Some things we just cannot do anything about, but if we are serious about healthy longevity, then this chapter is of vital importance. Overall health doesn't only refer to eating and exercising. There are many components to achieving optimum physical *and* mental health.

When we develop good habits and look after ourselves, then life really does get better in all areas. It goes back to motivation and forming the habits that need to become automatic in everyday life. You don't often, or maybe at all, hear a fit and healthy person complaining about being fit and healthy. Take this as an open secret, but also have some patience, and be realistic about the timeline of your health goals. I guess what we are about to consider are not really secrets but rather things we haven't yet thought about. Nonetheless, implementing them can be a relatively immediate goal, which will lead in time to your ultimate goal.

GIVE THE DEVICES A BREAK

We are attached to our electronic devices and carry laptops, cell phones, tablets, and the like around with us. Social media can be toxic, but we persist with it and the negativity it brings. Get into a habit of putting your phone down at 6 p.m. and only checking it again the next morning. Scrolling through Instagram until you fall asleep is bad for the sleep that will follow, bad for your eyes, and almost certainly bad for your self-esteem. Find a good book, go for a walk, be alone with your thoughts, and realign yourself.

Another thing about using your phone until you fall asleep is that it stimulates your brain. Even something as simple as sending a text to a friend and waiting for a response provides a stimulus that is counterproductive to sleep. Many of us are guilty of having our phones on our bedside table and checking them in the middle of the night. Even a quick glance can contribute to delayed sleep —if you are feeling tired during the day, you may now know what the solution is.

DEEP BREATHING EXERCISES

You know the drill—breathe in through your nose, and let your chest rise as you take in as much air as possible. Then let your chest fall as you release the breath through your mouth. The idea is relaxation, and everyone would rather feel relaxed than stressed. Finding a comfortable chair or lying down in an already relaxed position will be beneficial, and you can combine deep breathing with focusing on the present. Try to hold your inhale for 3 seconds and, when you exhale, do so slowly and rhyth-mically.

MINDFULNESS AND AWARENESS

Breathing exercises, as above, are part of mindfulness, and mindfulness is part of cognitive behavioral therapy. This is largely psychology based, but I am not going to go into this side of mindfulness. How to practice mindfulness is the important part, and mindfulness has been shown to have huge stress, worry, and anxiety avoidance benefits.

Breathing and Body Scanning

The section above on deep breathing exercises explains how to breathe, but not the mindfulness exercises you can use to accompany deep breathing. The first thing is to get into a comfortable position. Now here, breathing is not the essential part—don't forget to breathe, but pay more attention to what I am about to teach you as opposed to your breathing.

As you sit or lie in a comfortable position with your eyes closed, you must perform a body scan. Basically, this means paying deep attention to parts of your body as a distraction from your thoughts.

You can start by focusing on the top of your head. Take note of any sensations and, if you need to, pick out a point in your mind's eye and home in on it. Next, bring your attention to your ears. Picture them as you concentrate on any sounds you can hear. Touch your earlobes if you would like to and make a mental note of how they feel on your fingers. Then, focus on your nose as you breathe in deeply. Feel your nostrils expand as the air flows in. At the same time, observe the feeling of your chest rising. As you release the air, pay attention to what it feels like as it flows over your lips and your chest falls. Move down to your shoulders and move them slightly, as you experience how that feels. Follow this by focusing on your heartbeat, and accompany the feeling with a picture of your heart created in your mind.

I will stop at this point. I think you have enough information to do your own body scan. Be creative and do what makes you feel comfortable. The ultimate goal is a mind without thoughts and a completely relaxed body. It might sound a bit strange at first, but I recommend giving it a go before deciding whether or not it's for you.

Acute Awareness

If you talk to someone who has had a life-threatening illness, but has beaten it, they will undoubtedly tell you to make a point of appreciating the little things. Acute awareness calls on this principle, and is based on being present in the situation and paying deep attention to what it is that you are doing at the time. Let's say you decide to practice acute awareness while walking on the beach. Take time to look intensely at the ocean, how it moves, and the way the swell picks up gently and fades away. Notice the way the sea sweeps up over the sand and then retracts backwards, leaving the sand a different color. Take in the noise that the waves make, and the feeling of the salty breeze on your face. Dig your toes into the sand, close your eyes and face upward to feel the warm sun, then bring your gaze down to the horizon and focus on the furthest point you can see. Perhaps you want to get ankle deep in the water and enjoy the way it flows over your feet and toes. Try to eradicate any thoughts from your mind and only pay attention to the sensations you feel, the colors and things you see, the sounds you hear, and even the saltiness that you taste.

It isn't always easy to keep your mind completely absent of thought. However, if some form of worry or negativity creeps in, you must identify it, acknowledge its presence, and then usher it out of your mind as you refocus on what is happening in the moment.

Be Grateful

You get one life, and you should be grateful for it. If you are, then you will be more motivated to look after your weight and your general health. We all have things to be grateful for—remind yourself of what they are when you are struggling to get yourself off the couch and out for a jog. Be grateful for your body and for the chance to change your poor health habits. Be grateful for having the opportunity to get fit and to eat better. Be grateful for being able to cook instead of scrounging like so many people have been forced to do through circumstance. The more you focus on gratitude, the more likely you will be to make a change, find the motivation, and hang onto it.

WRITE IT DOWN

Firstly, use a pen and paper, not a computer. Keep a food diary and do calorie counts. Become obsessed and be proud of your progression toward a healthy diet. Don't leave anything out—you don't want to lie to yourself about a bar of chocolate you ate, for instance. Also, keep an exercise journal, where you set your fitness goals and monitor your progress. When you get into this habit and see your progress written down, it becomes more real, and your motivation to keep going will be on the up.

CHALLENGE YOURSELF

Getting out of your comfort zone in one area of life can have a positive impact on other areas. If you are dead set on getting healthy and losing weight, then look at alternatives to the traditional ideas of walking, jogging, or lifting weights. Join a tennis club or try out CrossFit. Do not challenge yourself only in health or weight loss-specific ways. Set yourself challenges at work, on a social level, to do with family relations—whatever will be a stretch to you. Having a goal or an objective will spill over into more goals and objectives.

GET THE RIGHT AMOUNT OF SLEEP

Sleep is more scientific than you might think. Sleep patterns, quality of sleep, and hours of sleep needed per day/night have been researched at length. In an article written for the Sleep Foundation website, based largely on study results, the following was put forward (Suni & Singh, 2023):

Knowing the general recommendations for how much sleep you need is a first step. Next, it is important to reflect on your individual needs based on factors like your activity level and overall health. And finally, of course, it is necessary to apply healthy sleep tips so you can actually get the full night's sleep that is recommended.

Furthermore, the writer offers a set of questions we can answer to determine how much sleep we need as individuals. The said questions are as follows:

- Are you productive, healthy, and happy on 7 hours of sleep? Or have you noticed you require more hours of sleep to get into high gear?
- Do you have coexisting health issues that might require more rest?
- Do you struggle to fall asleep? Do you wake up often during the night and struggle to get back to sleep?
- Do you experience anxiety when you are trying to fall asleep?

- Do you have a high level of daily energy expenditure? Do you frequently play sports or work in a labor-intensive job?
- Do your daily activities require alertness to do them safely? Do you drive every day and/or operate heavy machinery? Do you ever feel sleepy when doing these activities?
- Do you depend on caffeine to get you through the day?
- When you have an open schedule, do you tend to sleep later in the mornings?
- Are you experiencing a sleep disorder, or do you have a history of a sleep disorder? (Suni & Singh, 2023)

Not every question is relevant to every person, but you can see which questions are relevant to you. As per point three, labor-intensive jobs or sports will tire you out and can result in much better sleep. There is no better feeling than flopping into bed and, as the saying goes, "falling asleep as soon your head hits the pillow."

For the purposes of practicality, I am not going to go into every question. They are pretty self-explanatory. I will, however, put forward some sleep tips, followed by recommended sleep hours according to age.

Sleep Tips

- Stick to a set sleep schedule, within reason. Don't be too militant, but don't go to sleep at 2 a.m. one night (morning) and 9 p.m. the next night.
- Have a pre-bedtime routine and don't deviate from it unless you really have to.
- Do not consume caffeine or alcohol for several hours before going to bed.
- No devices—but you know this one already.
- Get rid of light or sound distractions. Blackout curtains and ear plugs will do the job.

Recommended Sleep Hours

- Infants: 12 to 16 hours
- Toddlers: 11 to 14 hours
- Preschool: 10 to 13 hours
- School age: 9 to 12 hours
- Teenagers: 8 to 10 hours
- Adults: 7 or more hours

It might be difficult to implement all of these tips and recommendations, but give it a good go and hopefully you can get into a healthy sleep routine to complement your health gains and weight loss. Putting new measures into practice is hardest to do in the beginning, but when you feel the benefits it will become something you *want* to keep doing.

LONGEVITY MYTHS

There are many misconceptions about what it takes to have a long and hopefully healthy life. We know what not to do, and the secrets in this chapter tell us what we should do. The catch is you don't want to live to be 85 if the last 10 years of your life are marred with sickness, ill health, and immobility as a result of your long-term obesity. It goes without saying that changes need to be made now, but, before we move on, it is still worthwhile to look at and get rid of some longevity myths.

Happy-Go-Lucky Equals a Long Life

Many believe that those people who are always smiling and joking around will live long and fulfilling lives. This is not the case, and a large reason for this is a lot of individuals put on figurative masks to hide pain and hardships. I realize this isn't diet or weight related, but you will notice people who may be overweight and obese have a self-deprecating attitude, but in a humorous way, to camouflage what is *really* going on.

Working Too Hard Makes You Die Young

It is not necessarily putting in long hours that contributes to ill-health, but rather the stress associated with work. It is quite possible to have an incredibly stressful job that only requires 30 hours a week. A huge source of stress is the "hurry up and wait" game. For instance, if your job involves coordinating imports and distributing the product, you may not have to work excessive hours, but the continuous stress worrying about goods arriving damaged, long delays, and letting down customers can contribute significantly to poor health. A quick tip—leave work at work! This can be tough to do indeed, but if you can get your mind off work stress, you are doing well... and exercise helps!

Genetics Dictates Life Span

This one does get onto the myth list because there is no conclusive study that has produced any concrete evidence on the topic. If your parents or grandparents died young, it doesn't mean you will too. The same applies to parents or grandparents who lived to older ages. The factors influencing life span are diverse. You may fall ill when you are young, or live with obesity, which none of your parents or grandparents lived with. In cases like this, longevity is unlikely, but when it comes down to it, genetics are not a genuine consideration.

Aging Is Terrible

Aging can be unpleasant—nobody wants to have aches and pains, or years of ill-health and immobility, but this is not always the case. Aging is largely circumstantial, and if you have aches and pains and are ill, then it can, and probably will, be an ongoing terrible experience. However, if you are happy and healthy in your old age, then it can be quite fun.

It Is Too Late to Correct Your Bad Habits

Giving up smoking, as an example, is going to be beneficial whether you are 20 or 80 years old. All you have to do is find the motivation and you can turn things around at any age. Most serious addicts never recover, but you can easily find stories of addicts who *have* recovered. Addiction is more than just bad habits—maybe try to find inspiration from someone who succumbed to addiction but clawed their way back.

CHAPTER SUMMARY

There are not really any secrets to overall health, just things you might not have thought about or investigated yet. However, giving your whole life an overhaul to become healthy in all areas is something within your grasp. Physical health is important, but so is mental health. Taking time out from electronic devices and social media is something of a mental cleanse. Deep breathing exercises work for many as a calming and relaxing tool, and the awareness you develop through mindfulness can assist in the same manner. Instead of rushing around and not appreciating small things like the warmth of the shower water and the beauty of nature, slow down and be present. Be grateful for what you have, make lists of the things you are grateful for, and challenge yourself to step out of your comfort zone.

Sleep is a great contributor to all-around good health. So, take note of the sleeping habits that can optimize good health. Implement a sleep schedule, and stick to it. Get into a "before bedtime" routine and sleep in a dark room with no distractions, and you will notice a general difference in your well-being.

Now you have the tools to look after your health, and not exclusively your weight, I hope you have learned the required lessons to lead an overall healthy life. However, in terms of weight loss specifically, you need to keep it off. In the next chapter we will look at how to do so.

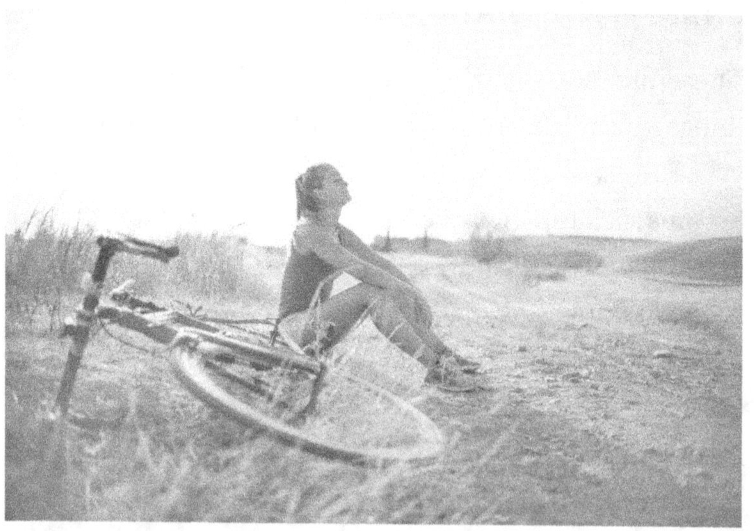

7

MANAGING YOUR WEIGHT

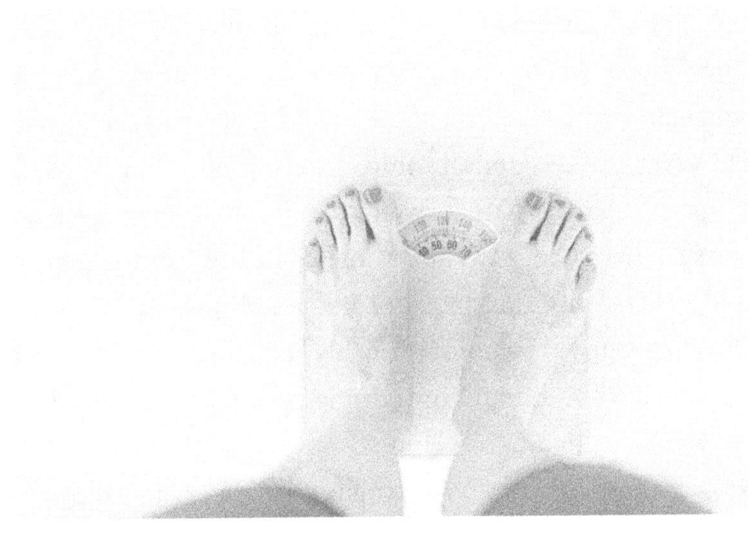

Several of the studies I have referred to point to diets not working, but when you do weight loss the healthy way, then there is a much greater chance of keeping it off. The answer is relatively simple—maintain your healthy lifestyle. Making the changes needed to lose weight are long-term changes. As time goes by, your good lifestyle choices and the practice thereof become good habits. You may need to refocus from time to time and get back on track, but maintenance and consistency are what you should be aiming for. There is a bit more to it than this, and I realize challenges may arise, so we need to delve a bit deeper. With a greater understanding of weight management and/or maintenance, the task becomes a little more simple.

WHAT EXACTLY IS WEIGHT MANAGEMENT?

You should remember the BMI section, which gave guidelines as to weight and its classifications (underweight, normal, overweight, obese, and morbidly obese). However, there is no absolutely definitive way of classifying someone as underweight, normal, overweight, or obese. This is because our bodies all differ, some greatly and others only slightly. A professional middle- or long-distance runner would probably be classed as underweight, but the amount of training they engage in explains why it is difficult for them to put on weight (I am not saying these athletes want to gain weight—this would be counterproductive to their purposes). In addition, middle- and long-distance runners need to be lean—the less they weigh, the more streamlined they are. A heavyweight boxer could be said to be overweight, but they need to weigh a significant amount to be competitive in the ring. Also, remember these two extremes—middle- and long-distance runners, and boxers—monitor, manage, and maintain their weight differently.

In addition to BMI, there are waist-size recommendations, but they are nothing more than recommendations, for the same reasons as in the previous paragraph. As a matter of interest, women are said to have a recommended waist circumference of 35 inches, and men should measure up at 40 inches (WebMD Editorial Contributors, 2021). These numbers are not hard and fast rules, but they act as guidelines.

The point is to reach *your* ideal weight, not the weight of a runner, boxer, celebrity, or friend. When you reach your ideal weight, you need to manage it through healthy eating and exercise. This applies equally whether you are underweight, overweight, or obese—not in the sense of the methods you will use, but in the need to maintain your ideal weight once you have reached it.

So, to answer the question in simple terms: Weight management is managing your ideal weight after you attain it, on an ongoing and hopefully everlasting basis.

EXERCISE FOR WEIGHT LOSS AND MANAGEMENT

I am not sure if you recall that your BMR is about two-thirds of the total calories burned. So, with better eating and exercise, your calorie-burning ability will be enhanced. What do I mean? If you are eating better, this will reduce your calorie intake, and adding exercise will burn calories you were not previously burning through exercise. So, essentially, you are hitting weight loss from all angles: via a reduction of intake as well as an increase in calories burned.

There is a plethora of information around about what the best type of exercise is. The fact is, however, there is no "best" exercise. You need to find something suited to you, and even though you may see exercise as a chore, you can find a routine that feels like the least bad chore. But exercise can be fun, and the fitter you get the more fun it becomes. Doing three push-ups might sound like an arduous and unpleasant task now, but when you can do 10, then three will seem easy… slowly, slowly catch the weight-maintenance monkey! Here are a few suggestions, from simple to slightly complicated ones, which you could take up as weight-management exercises.

Walking

Start off with 30 minutes on Monday, Wednesday, and Friday. This way, you are giving your body some time to recover, which is vital. You will feel some stiffness at first, which is why you need to have a day or more to allow your body to recover. However, with time your body will get more accustomed to the exertion, and as you become more comfortable after exercising, you can increase your frequency to four times a week and your duration to 45 minutes per session, and so on. In 2014, a 12-week walking study with obese subjects saw the participants walk for between 50 and 70 minutes three times per week. The average weight loss noted was 1.5% of total body weight. Waist-circumference reduction averaged out at 2.8 centimeters (just over 1 inch) (Hong et al, 2014).

There are many studies like this, and there is no doubt walking is a great way to lose weight and maintain your desired weight.

Running or Jogging

Running requires more exertion than walking, which means running or jogging for the same amount of time as walking will result in more calorie shedding. If you want to transition from walking to running, you can do so slowly. Walking for 10 minutes, then running for 5, then repeating until you hit your time goal is a good way to transition. Otherwise, you can walk on one day, run on the next, and continue to alternate your days. We will get to interval training, but very quickly, there is a type of running training called "fartlek."

Fartlek

Fartlek mixes up running speeds and intensities. So, you might run 2 miles at a fast pace, followed by half a mile really slowly. Then you could get into a fast/slow pattern, where you run at sprinting pace until you can't keep it up anymore. At this point you slow down to a pace just faster than a walk until you feel 90% recovered, and then you hit the next sprint.

You can go out for a run without a specific plan, and improvise as you go. Perhaps you would like to up your pace for the distance between lampposts, then reduce it for double that distance, then repeat. You could push your speed when running up hills and slow it right down when you descend. Use your imagination and creativity, which could also alleviate some of the mundanity of running. This is the type of training you can tailor to the way you feel on the day, and it is used by many world-class middle- and long-distance athletes.

Cycling

The first advantage of cycling is there is very little impact on your joints when riding a bicycle. If you don't want to cycle outdoors, you have the stationary bike option at the gym, or you can pick one up for home use. If you are going to try cycling, you will want to ride for anywhere between an hour and 90 minutes. Three to four times a week should be good at first; however, an increase in frequency will do no harm.

Cycling also gives you options, and trail cycling or mountain biking is becoming increasingly popular, with mountain bike clubs popping up all over the place. If you like to get outdoors while burning calories then a mountain bike may be a good purchase.

Weight Training

If you intend to get into weight training, it would be best to consult a professional to design a program tailored specifically for you. If you don't know what you are doing, then you risk injury, which could become a huge setback to your whole exercise plan. There have been extensive studies into weight training and metabolism. The results may inspire you to get into weights as opposed to walking, jogging, or cycling.

A study performed over 24 weeks found young men who engaged in weight training saw a 9% increase in their metabolic rate, and young women were able to note an increase of 4%. Those percentages equate to 140 extra calories per day for the men and 50 extra for the women (Lemmer et al., 2001).

Mixing weight training and cardio training like walking, running, or cycling has even greater impacts on weight loss and maintenance. Perhaps combining weight training with cardio should be your goal!

Interval Training

If you are not used to exercise and want to get it over with as quickly as possible, then interval training might be for you. It is characterized by short bursts of intense activity, followed by periods of rest/recovery. Because of the intensity, you can spend less time working out and burn the same amount of calories as you would on a longer run or walk. As an example, you could pedal as fast as you can on a stationary bike for 30 seconds, then pedal at a slow and comfortable rate for 1 minute, and repeat. Only 10 to 30 minutes in total are needed. This is the type of training where you spend more time recovering because of the sheer intensity of your exertion, whatever it may be.

Swimming

Breaststroke burns the most calories, followed by butterfly, backstroke, and freestyle. Swimming causes virtually zero impact, so there is no strain on your joints and, as a result, minimal chance of injury. An often quoted 12-week study into middle-aged women found three 60-minute swimming sessions per week significantly decreased their body fat, and additionally improved flexibility and reduced risk of heart disease (Lee & Oh, 2015).

Similar to fartlek running, you can mix up your swimming speeds and/or effort levels. As a suggestion, you can do one lap fast, then walk the length of the pool very slowly, and repeat. There will be mild resistance as you take steps through the water, so even if you are only making ground slowly, you are still engaging in a mild form of exertion. Alternating strokes to work different muscle groups is also recommended. Water aerobics is a form of swimming, you could say. Classes are available at most gyms with pools, and even though the calorie-burning benefits are not as high as they are with swimming, you will definitely have some low-impact fun.

Yoga

If you are also aiming for increased flexibility, yoga could be your go-to. A study into yoga and obesity found just two yoga sessions per week, at 90 minutes per session, resulted in waist measurement reductions of approximately 3.8 centimeters (around 1.5 inches) (Crameret al., 2016).

Yoga is also said to be good for focus and mental health, in addition to the social element. Also, you will notice many yoga studios have little cafés attached that sell healthy food, which is a convenient benefit.

Believe it or not, there are 15 different types of yoga, including the most well-known, which is called Hatha yoga. Within the different types of yoga there are a variety of poses, and yoga teachers will have no problem with you leaving some of them out if they are difficult at first.

Pilates

Although Pilates and yoga are not the same, many similarities exist, as they are both largely stretching based. Pilates does not burn as many calories as running or swimming, but its popularity indicates that people enjoy it and stick with it for the long term. Most gyms offer Pilates classes, and they generally range from an hour to 90 minutes. You should aim for three times a week at first, and, if you enjoy the classes, then up your frequency to four times per week. Like yoga, there is also a social element. If you enjoy the actual exercises and you make some new friends, then you are winning in two areas.

Other

You can get creative with exercising and make things more fun, and possibly more adventurous. You could fill two buckets with water and carry them around your garden, or do shuttle runs, star jumps, and burpees. You could even walk up and down your stairs. I would also recommend checking out some YouTube videos on alternative exercising. A quick tip: If you drive to get groceries, park your car in the furthest parking space from the store. You are then killing two birds with one stone by burning some extra calories walking to and from your car, as well as getting your shopping done.

A growing sport in the United States is called pickleball. Chances are you have heard of it, but if not, pickleball is a combination of elements of tennis, squash, and badminton. It is a lot of fun and is great for weight loss and weight management. While you are on YouTube finding out about alternative exercises, watch a few videos on pickleball. It is played by all ages, and the pickleball community is very welcoming. If you enjoy the game, then exercising while playing will not feel like a chore at all.

Don't rule out getting involved in some social team sports like soccer, softball, volleyball, or even ultimate frisbee. These activities do require a certain amount of mobility, but don't get discouraged—think back to the section on chair exercises and my advice to shed weight until you are comfortable walking for 1 km, at which point you can supplement chair workouts with the types of exercise discussed above.

Here are a couple of additional tips to help you think outside the box and throw in some calorie-burning activities during the non-exercising parts of your day:

- Take the stairs as opposed to the elevator. You are then killing two birds with one stone by burning some extra calories walking up the stairs, as well as getting to where you need to be.
- If you have a desk job and you have to get up from time to time to go to the printer or to attend

meetings, then make the walks to and from those events brisk. Take the stairs instead of the elevator, and take the scenic route when you can.

WHY SHOULD YOU BOTHER?

It sounds like a defeatist question, but other than the irrefutable health benefits, there are other areas in your life that will benefit from you maintaining your ideal weight. An interesting article published on the Southside Medical website explains that studies have shown people who are overweight to be less likely to succeed in the workplace, and many patients struggling with obesity also experience mental-health disorders like anxiety and depression. Because patients with weight issues often can't participate in regular activities, they experience distress and are worried about missing out.

Put simply, the results of studies like these point to happiness and a more fulfilling life if you lose weight and maintain your weight loss—which is why you should definitely bother. Keep this in mind when you feel like you are getting nowhere!

You should also bother because you need to see your health as a priority. If you are working remotely, it means you are at an elevated risk level when it comes to putting on weight. In general, we don't move around enough, and even if you don't work remotely, there is still a high chance you would put on weight if you drove to work or were driven there. Twenty-first-century life lends itself to increased obesity—we know this well, but nevertheless we still succumb to unhealthy lifestyles.

COMPLICATIONS

This is another reason why we should bother. Underlying diseases can be better managed by weight maintenance or can have their onset delayed. Type 2 diabetes is a classic example, and studies have shown excess body weight to be associated with the risk of cardiometabolic complications, which are major causes of morbidity and mortality in type 2 diabetes (Wilding, 2014).

Prediabetic individuals who lose weight significantly delay the onset of the disease. Weight loss improves glycemic control and, when combined with major calorie restriction, it can reverse the progression of type 2 diabetes. Unfortunately, the same study revealed "weight loss interventions did not reduce the rate of cardiovascular events in overweight or obese adults with type 2 diabetes," but on a positive note, weight loss interventions "include improvements in quality of life, mobility, and physical and sexual function" (Wilding, 2014).

Obviously, there are many other health complications associated with obesity, and a study published in the journal *Therapeutic Advances in Endocrinology and Metabolism* makes this patently clear. Not only are the complications a major health risk themselves, but the frequency thereof is putting the United States' national health-care system under severe strain (Ansari, 2022).

Anatomical Effects

You may remember in Chapter 2 we dealt with adipose tissue; to jog your memory, this is fatty tissue in your body that places strain on different parts of the body. In obese people, an excess amount of adipose tissue can lead to sleep apnea, as mentioned previously. Other risks include obesity hypoventilation syndrome and gastroesophageal reflux disease.

Obesity hypoventilation syndrome is also called Pickwickian syndrome. The disorder is breathing related and affects some people who have obesity. What happens is your blood is occupied by an excess amount of carbon dioxide, which means there is not enough space for oxygen. This occurs due to hypoventilation, which means breathing at an abnormally slow rate.

Below is a list of the symptoms:

- shortness of breath
- ongoing fatigue
- lack of energy
- daytime sluggishness
- headaches and neck pain
- dizziness
- depression and anxiety

- loud and persistent snoring
- choking or gasping when you are asleep
- pauses in breathing while asleep

Gastroesophageal reflux disease is a particularly dangerous, and very unpleasant, illness where stomach acid repeatedly flows back into the esophagus, which connects your mouth and stomach. This creates acid reflux, which can irritate the lining of your esophagus and is marked by the following symptoms:

- a burning sensation in your chest (heartburn), usually after eating, which might be worse at night or when lying down
- acid reflux
- backwash (regurgitation) of food or sour liquid
- upper abdominal or chest pain
- trouble swallowing, even when drinking water (dysphagia)
- sensation of a lump in your throat or feeling as if something is stuck in your throat
- an ongoing cough
- inflammation of the vocal cords (laryngitis)
- new or worsening asthma

It is not possible to go into every condition; however, the information in Chapter 2, along with the above and what you will learn below, pretty much encapsulates the extent of the negative effects on your health as an obese individual.

Metabolic Effects

The impact of obesity on metabolism is not less or more important than its anatomical effects and is most certainly worthy of serious attention. The metabolism-influencing guilty party in the adipose tissue is proinflammatory cytokines. To the nonscientific, including myself, you get pro- and anti-inflammatory cytokines; here, we are concerned with the proinflammatory type. Cytokines are proteins released by cells, and in obese individuals excess secretion can result in nonalcoholic fatty liver disease, insulin resistance, and cardiovascular disease.

KNOW YOUR STUFF

I am sure by this point you have learned a whole bunch of new things. This is great, but I want you to understand the reasons why so many people regain weight and how to avoid this trap. Johns Hopkins Medicine (n.d.) explains the crux of the matter as follows:

While losing weight is difficult for many people, it is even more challenging to keep the weight off. Most people who lose a large amount of weight have regained it two to three years later. One theory about regaining lost weight is that people who decrease the amount of calories they consume to lose weight experience a drop in the rate their bodies burn calories. This makes it increasingly difficult to lose weight over a period of months. A lower rate of burning calories may also make it easier to regain weight after a more normal diet is resumed. For these reasons, extremely low-calorie diets and rapid weight loss are discouraged.

The recommendation is to consult a nutritionist, who will probably advise a test-type approach. It is generally accepted that to test your body's ability to keep the weight off after achieving your desired weight, you should add a small amount of calories daily—200 is a good amount. You want to closely monitor the effect on your weight. If you are still losing weight, then you have to up your calorie intake per day. The ideal "test" period is 1 week. If you put on weight in the test period, then you need to adjust your calorie intake or increase calorie-burning activities.

It is also a good idea to learn more about calories and perhaps download a calorie-counting app, so you can monitor your intake. It can actually become quite addictive because you can start making accurate predictions in a more informed way. If you go to Healthline, you can find an evaluation and rating of some weight-loss and calorie-counting apps (Gunners, 2019), but MyFitnessPal is probably the most well-known and frequently used one. You can actually even Google how many calories are in whatever food or drink, and while the accuracy cannot be guaranteed, a ballpark figure will be just fine.

The more you find out about nutrition, calories, kilojoules, and what you are putting into your body, the more you will want to know. Imagine if I told you leading a healthy lifestyle would lower your risk of illness, make you happier, make life easier in general, elevate your self-esteem, and make you a more confident, well-rounded individual—you would lose weight and be healthy, right? Well, I speak only the truth, and the rest is up to you.

CHAPTER SUMMARY

Once you have lost the weight, you don't want to pile it back on, so you have to engage in weight management. This would involve aiming at staying within the healthy BMI range (this is, of course, dependent on your height, but you are looking at a target BMI of between 25 and 35), and having a waist circumference of 35 inches for women and 45 inches for men. There are different ideal weights for different people—remember, a boxer is different from a runner.

Exercise is a vital part of weight management, and there are various types of exercises you can do. On the one hand, you have the traditional walking, running, swimming, and cycling. On the other, you have the alternative varieties that yoga and Pilates provide, and of course, weight training and interval training. Team sports can be a great way of socializing and having fun while you maintain your ideal weight. You can consider soccer, softball, volleyball, and basically anything you think will be enjoyable.

You should avoid the "why bother" attitude for many reasons, but a particularly important one is to prevent or reduce the complications and risks of being overweight or obese. Maintaining and managing your weight can subdue underlying diseases or delay their onset, whether anatomic or metabolic. Otherwise, learning more about calories and counting them will be beneficial in losing, maintaining, and managing your weight.

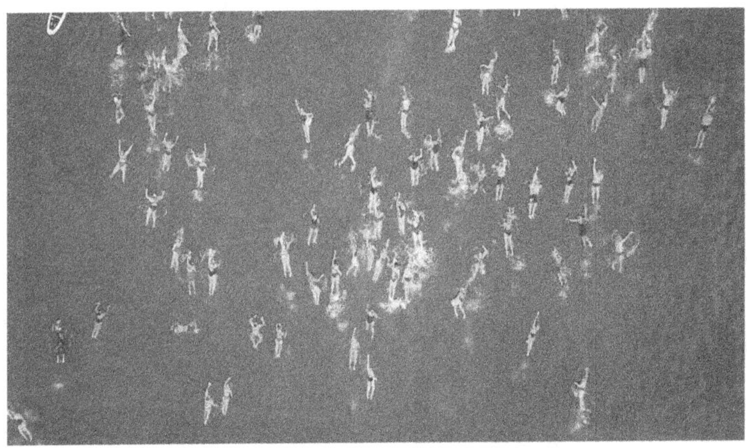

CONCLUSION

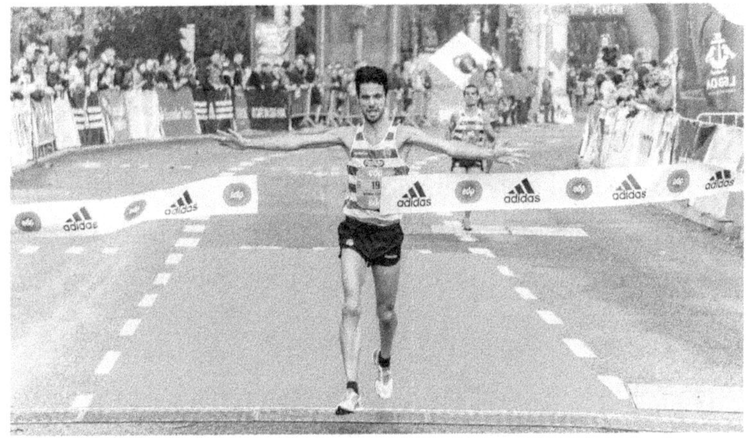

So, here we are at the end of this life-changing book—I hope you have started implementing what you have learned. Or at least, I hope you have found the inspiration to begin implementation. Unless you are afflicted with the metabolism-affecting diseases discussed, then there is no excuse not to get healthy. Even if you do have metabolic syndrome, improving your health can have no negative ramifications. You *can* do it, but you really have to *want* to do it before you will roll your sleeves up, take action, and turn the persistent and unhealthy negatives into ongoing healthy positives.

Some of my further hopes are that you have taken note of the statistics and are alarmed by them. If things keep progressing the way they are, we are going to be staring down a barrel where more people are obese and overweight than are a healthy weight. It is not only about turning a corner yourself, but getting others to do so as well. I was able to turn my life around and become perpetually fit and healthy. If I can do it, then so can you. Don't wait until you are confined to a wheelchair before you try to make a change. Take stock of how you feel generally and what you look like, and decide whether you like it—from then, it is up to you, but I do believe you can get healthy!

What follows will act as a concise summary of the most important parts of the book, chronologically. The reason for this is to give you necessary reminders of what you need to focus on, but also to facilitate an easy way to refer back to particular sections you may want to revisit, and to be used as a "power play" of motivation.

We know there is an overweight and obesity epidemic, and we know the fundamental cause is an imbalance in calories consumed versus calories burned. The consequences can be devastating, and are likely to bring on premature illness and, very possibly, early death—we do not want this!

Let me remind you about malnutrition, covered in Chapter 1, which does not only mean undereating. The crux is the lack of necessary nutrients. Even if you overeat on a daily basis, if *what* you are eating does not contain the nutrients you require to function in a healthy manner, then you too will suffer from malnutrition. Smoking, and to a larger degree excess alcohol intake, only worsen the situation and accelerate the onset of diseases and illnesses in a "double whammy" kind of way.

If you happen to be older and obese, you are in a way lucky to have made it this far, but it is not too late to make changes. Obesity in children and adolescents is concerningly on the rise, and parents are essentially to blame. Sadly, race and ethnicity are linked to obesity because of the socioeconomic position in which marginalized communities find themselves. Social services, grants, and welfare initiatives need to be stepped up. The following fact remains true: The less money you have, the cheaper the food is that you can purchase, and cheap food is generally lacking in the health department. There are minor genetic factors, but obesogenic issues, such as environment and access to healthy foods, play a bigger part. Mental health is affected by obesity, and vice versa. Obese individuals often become anxious or depressed as a result of their negative self-image and inability to lead a healthy life. Depressed individuals often lack the serotonin necessary to create motivation to exercise, and, combined with self-medication via eating and drinking, the result is often obesity.

As covered in Chapter 2, BMI is a person's weight divided by the square of their height. A high BMI can indicate high body fatness. BMI screens for weight categories that may lead to health problems, but it does not diagnose the health of an individual. Even though BMI doesn't hold absolute accuracy in the same way as a blood test for high blood pressure, the indication of health problems is pretty on point. You can refer back to Chapter 2 for the details of healthy weight classifications as informed by BMI.

Adiposity is the excess buildup of fatty tissue. It starts growing around the age of 1 year and stops around 7 years of age. Adiposity rebound denotes BMI increase and fat increase after the decline. Adiposity rebound can be a predictor of later obesity.

High blood pressure is worryingly common in overweight and obese individuals and can be a contributing factor to arrhythmia, cardiomyopathy, coronary heart disease, and heart failure. Further ramifications include strokes and heart attacks, among other dangers. The details of the aforesaid can be found in Chapter 2. The list of adverse conditions where being overweight or obese leads to a heightened risk is not quite endless; however, it is certainly long. Clustering of lifestyle factors, which is a combination of poor health choices, only makes long-term health prospects worse—the four most common combination indulgences are smoking, excessive alcohol intake, lack of exercise, and lack of vegetable and fruit intake.

At the risk of repeating myself, but out of necessity to do so, we know diets don't work, but there are many myths about diet-related subjects. Despite popular belief, calories differ. They have the same energy content, but act differently as foods go through different internal passageways. Carbohydrates don't necessarily make you fat—*excess consumption* of carbs is what makes you gain weight. Other myths are supplements cause weight loss, eating fat makes you fat, and diets work.

Metabolism is constituted by chemical interactions at a cellular level, and comprises catabolism and anabolism, as we learnt in Chapter 3. The former is concerned with breaking down food components. The latter takes care of cell growth, energy storage, and tissue maintenance. They work together as instructed by the nervous system and hormonal system. Part of it is the BMR, which describes the kilojoules your body burns when it is at rest. Then there is the energy consumption used during exercise or exertion, plus the thermic effect, being the amount of energy used to eat, digest, and metabolize food.

Fasting can be a contentious topic, but it has the potential to work if it is done consistently. The three most popular methods of fasting are alternate day, whole day, and time restricted. However, there is no clear evidence suggesting these methods are superior in any way when it comes to weight loss. Ideally, we should stay away from fasting and get the balance we all know of into action.

The 7-day eating plan is one you should refer back to, but to give you a reminder, it consists of five meals per day over a 7-day period, which should be repeated as a long-term lifestyle intervention. The five meals are breakfast, morning snack, lunch, afternoon snack, and dinner. As I said in Chapter 4, don't be afraid to get creative. I also encourage you to look at the recipe websites I listed at the end of Chapter 4, and consider buying one of the best-selling cookbooks I referred to.

Metabolic disorders are an unfortunate reality. They are genetic and often incurable, but they can be managed to some degree through healthy eating and exercise. Symptoms of some of the disorders include stomach aches, enlarged organs, liver damage, severely depleted energy, breathing problems, and a whole host of others across the spectrum of metabolic disorders.

Weight cycling or yo-yo dieting is when individuals jump from diet to diet, causing weight fluctuation. Most often a little bit of weight is lost and all of it put back on, plus more. This is strongly advised against, and with the right motivation you can develop the healthy lifestyle you desire. Try to develop a support network and people to hold you accountable, to use as extra motivational tools. If you have an exercise partner or join an exercise group, then you can draw motivation from the need to avoid letting these people down.

Diets remain a mystery and when people tell you diets make you fat, it is not so much the specific diet, but rather the bounce back after having completed the diet. The studies discussed in Chapter 5 provide concrete evidence diets really do not work, at least for most of those who try them. It is all about healthy choices that can be sustained, as well as mindful eating—i.e., really deeply focusing on the eating experience—and of course, exercise.

There are no secrets to good health, per se, but putting certain measures into practice can improve overall health. Cutting down on electronic devices and engaging in relaxing behavior like deep breathing and mindfulness can help you to find more balance, and you can refer back to Chapter 6 in this regard. Be grateful for what you have and acknowledge those things—writing them down acts as a visceral motivator. Set yourself challenges and make sure you get *good* sleep, which involves the right number of hours without distraction.

As mentioned previously, it is not only about losing weight and becoming healthy, but also about maintenance when you reach your ideal body weight. As discussed in

Chapter 7, we all have different ideal weights and you need to acknowledge what yours is. Healthy eating must continue, along with exercise, to allow you to manage your weight. In terms of exercise, walking, running or swimming for 30 minutes three times a week initially, building up to longer durations and greater frequency over time, are very effective for weight maintenance. Cycling offers the same benefits; however, longer sessions are required, at 1 hour to 90 minutes. Weight training, after advice from a professional, offers weight maintenance as a non-cardio activity, and high-intensity interval training allows for shorter sessions. Yoga and Pilates have grown in popularity and studios are abundant, plus there is a social element if you want to make new friends (a great idea to garner some accountability).

At the end of the day it still comes down to your motivation. The fact is, in order to lose weight you need to burn more calories than you ingest. It is simple to write it down or say it out loud, but the implementation is the difficult bit. You can do it—I wholeheartedly believe you can, and so should you, as well as the people who form your support system.

I would love to hear your stories about success in weight loss, healthy eating, and exercise, in addition to continued maintenance and management. It would be a great help if you could leave a review and if you wish, some comments.

I will leave you with a quote from Nelson Mandela, Nobel Peace Prize winner—"It always seems impossible until it's done"—and my final word: Get out there, and get it done! Things will get tough, but you are resilient and you can do this! Believe in yourself… always!

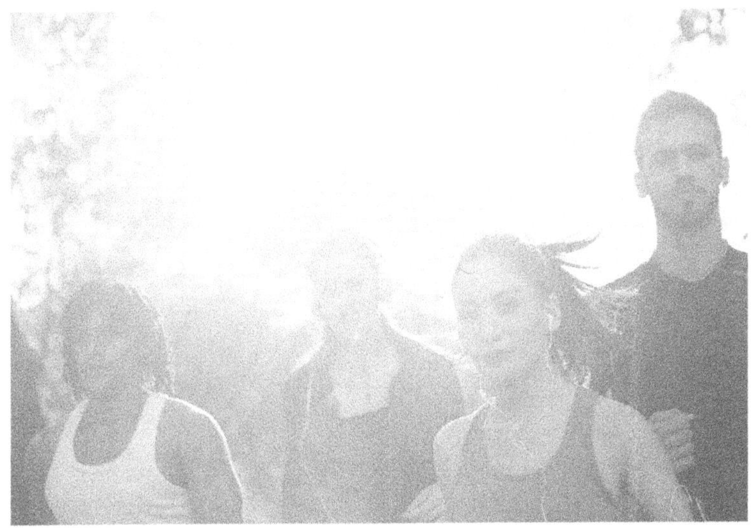

GLOSSARY

- **Adiposity:** Too much fatty tissue in the body.
- **Anabolism:** The growth of new cells, the storage of energy, and the maintenance of body tissues are all taken care of by anabolism.
- **Atwater factors:** One gram of fat contains 9 calories, while one gram of protein or carbohydrates contains 4 calories. Wilber O. Atawar discovered this in 1890, and thus the numbers became known as the "Atwater factors."
- **BMI:** Body mass index, calculated as weight (in kilograms) divided by height (in meters and centimeters) squared. BMI levels are indicators of obesity and potentially associated health conditions.
- **Calories:** A unit of measurement telling us how much energy is in a particular food or drink.

- **Catabolism:** Breaking down of proteins, carbohydrates, and fats to produce cellular activity through energy.
- **Glucose:** Part of the carbohydrate group called "simple sugars," and a source of energy for the body.
- **Noncommunicable diseases:** Diseases that are not spread through viruses or infection.
- **Musculoskeletal disorders:** Diseases that affect the muscles and the skeleton, i.e., ligaments, bones, joints, muscles, and tendons.
- **Obesogenic:** An amalgamation of the words "obese" and "genetic." Obesogenic factors have the potential to lead to obesity.

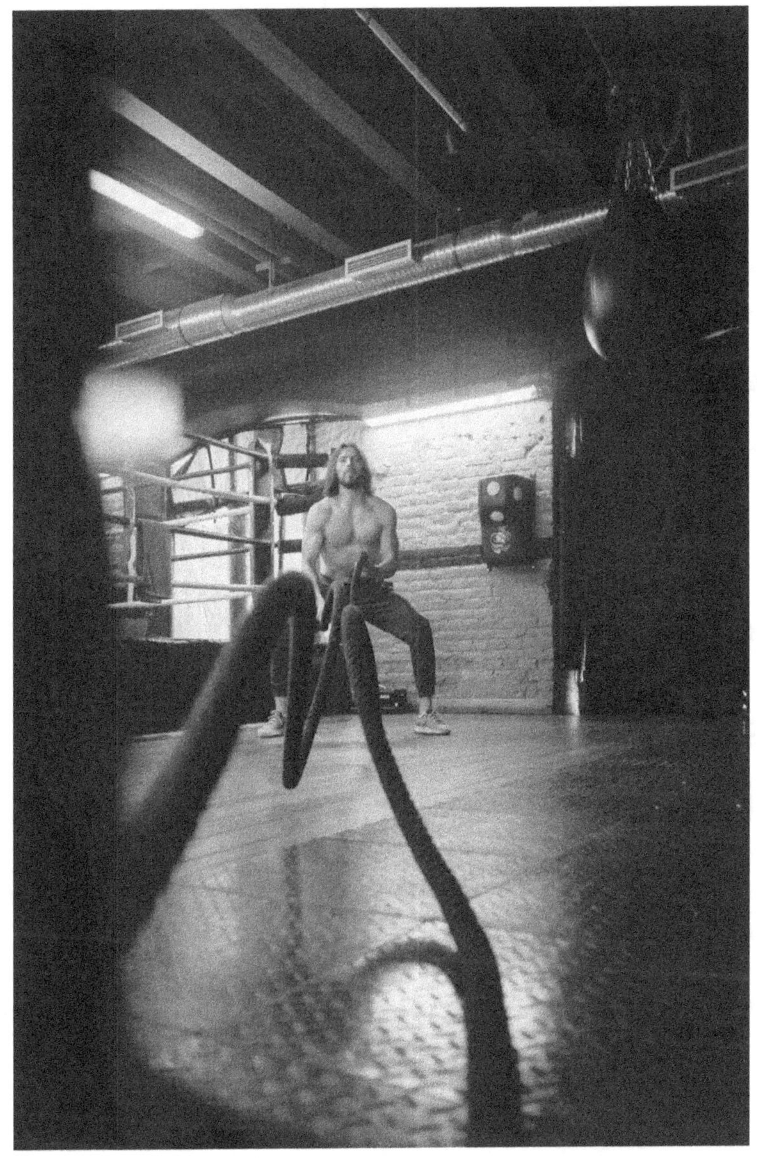

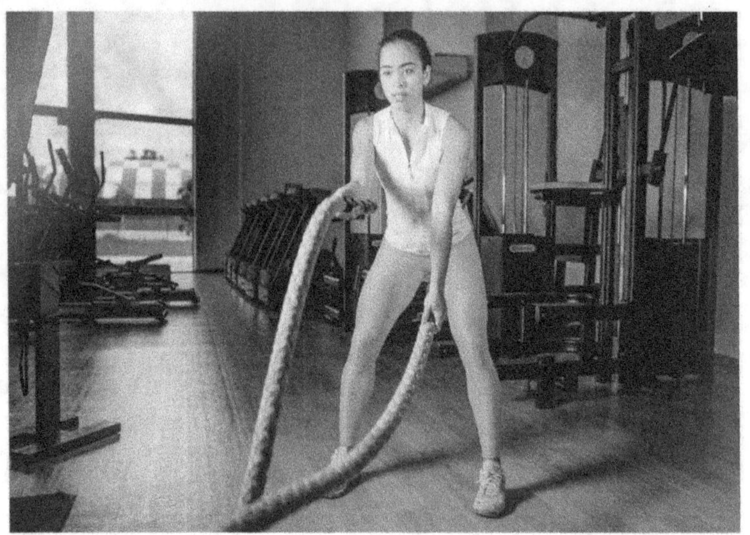

REFERENCES

Alcohol and weight gain. (n.d.). Better Health Channel. https://www.betterhealth.vic.gov.au/health/healthyliving/Alcohol-and-weight-gain

Allison, M. B., & Myers Jr, M. G. (2014). 20 years of leptin: connecting leptin signaling to biological function. *Journal of Endocrinology, 223*(1), 25-35.

American Heart Association. (2022, December 5). *Warning signs of a heart attack.* https://www.heart.org/en/health-topics/heart-attack/warning-signs-of-a-heart-attack

Annie E. Casey Foundation. (2021, September 2o). *New child poverty data illustrate the powerful impact of America's safety net programs.* https://www.aecf.org/blog/new-child-poverty-data-illustrates-the-powerful-impact-of-americas-safety-net-programs

Ansari, S., Haboubi, H., & Haboubi, N. (2020). Adult obesity complications: Challenges and clinical impact. *Therapeutic Advances in Endocrinology and Metabolism, 11,* 2042018820934955.

Aronoff, J.E., Ragin, A., Wu, C., Markl, M., Schnell, S., Shaibani, A., Blaire, C., & Kuzawa, CW. (2022). Why do humans undergo an adiposity rebound? Exploring links with the energetic costs of brain development in childhood using MRI-based 4D measures of total cerebral blood flow. *International Journal of Obesity, 46,* 1044-1050.

Armitage, J. A., Poston, L., & Taylor, P. (2008). Developmental origins of obesity and the metabolic syndrome: The role of maternal obesity. *Frontiers of Hormone Research, 36,* 73–84.

Ayrton, A. (2021, January 20). Thoughtful woman choosing between green apple and sweet donut. [Picture]. Pexels. https://www.pexels.com/photo/thoughtful-woman-choosing-between-green-apple-and-sweet-donut-6550797/

Baer, D. J., & Novoty, J. A. (2018). Metabolizable energy from cashew nuts is less than that predicted by Atwater factors. *Nutrients, 11*(1), 33.

Bariatric surgery risks, complications, and side effects. (n.d.). UPMC. https://www.upmc.com/services/bariatrics/candidate/risks-and-complications

Basal metabolic rate calculator. (2016, July 1). Garnet Health. https://www.garnethealth.org/news/basal-metabolic-rate-calculator

Berkley, B. (2022, April 21). *Diet culture: A brief history.* https://sahrc.org/2022/04/diet-culture-a-brief-history/

Calories burned shopping: Calculator and formula. (2020, September 24). Captain Calculator. https://captaincalculator.com/health/calorie/calories-burned-shopping-calculator/

Cameron, N., & Demerath, E. W. (2002). Critical periods in human growth and their relationship to diseases of aging. *American Journal of Physical Anthropology, 40,* 159–184.

Caplan, Z., & Rabe, M. (2023, May 25). *The older population: 2020.* https://www.census.gov/library/publications/2023/decennial/c2020br-07.html

Centers for Disease Control and Prevention. (2021, May 18). *High blood pressure symptoms and causes.* https://www.cdc.gov/bloodpressure/about.htm

Centers for Disease Control and Prevention. (2022, May 17). *Childhood obesity facts.* https://www.cdc.gov/obesity/data/childhood.html

Centers for Disease Control and Prevention. (2022, June 3). *Body mass index (BMI).* https://www.cdc.gov/healthyweight/assessing/bmi/index.html

Centers for Disease Control and Prevention. (2023, May 4). *Current cigarette smoking among adults in the United States.* https://www.cdc.gov/tobacco/data_statistics/fact_sheets/adult_data/cig_smoking/index.htm

Centers for Disease Control and Prevention. (2023, June 28). *Finding a balance of food and activity.* https://www.cdc.gov/healthyweight/calories/other_factors.html

Chatkin, R., Mottin, C. C., & Chatkin, J. M. (2010). Smoking among morbidly obese patients. *BMC Pulmonary Medicine Journal 10,* 61.

Cleveland Clinic. (2021, August 30). *Metabolism.* https://my.clevelandclinic.org/health/body/21893-metabolism

Cleveland Clinic. (2022, October 27). *Obesity hypoventilation syndrome.* https://my.clevelandclinic.org/health/diseases/24393-obesity-hypoventilation-syndrome

Cleveland Clinic. (2023, June 26). *11 ways to spot a fad diet.* https://my.clevelandclinic.org/health/articles/9476-fad-diets

Cramer, H., Thoms, M. S., Annheyer, D., Lauche, R., & Dobos, G. (2016). Yoga in women with abdominal obesity—a randomized controlled trial. *Deutsches Ärzteblatt International, 113*(39), 645–652.

Dachis, A. (2011, October 26). *"It always seems impossible until it is done."* Lifehacker. https://lifehacker.com/it-always-seems-impossible-until-it-is-done-5853601

De Brabandere, S. (2017, March 16). *Human body ratios: A project that measures up.* Scientific American. https://www.scientificamerican.com/article/human-body-ratios/

Diet review: Intermittent fasting for weight loss. (n.d.) Harvard T. H. Chan School of Public Health. https://www.hsph.harvard.edu/nutritionsource/healthy-weight/diet-reviews/intermittent-fasting/

Dolgoff, S. (2021, March 6). *Stop believing these longevity myths to live a longer, healthier, and happier life.* Prevention. https://www.prevention.com/health/a35217718/longevity-myths/

Dulloo, A. G., & Montani, J.-P. (2015). Pathways from dieting to weight regain, to obesity, and to the metabolic syndrome: An overview. *The Obesity Review Journal, 16*(Suppl. 1), 1–6

Finkelstein, E. A., & Kruger, E. (2014, June 24). Meta- and cost-effectiveness analysis of commercial weight loss strategies. *Obesity, 22*(9), 1942–1951.

Foster, G. D., Wadden, T. A., Kendall, P. C., Sunkard, A. J., & Vogt, R. A. (1996). Psychological effects of weight loss and regain: a prospective evaluation. *Journal of Consulting and Clinical Pschology, 64*(4), 752–757.

Gearhardt, A,. Singer, D., Kirch, M., Solway, E., Roberts, S., Smith, E., Hutchens, L., Malani, P., & Kullgren, J. (2023, January/February). *Addiction to highly processed food among older adults.* University of Michigan National Poll on Healthy Aging. https://www.healthyagingpoll.org/reports-more/report/addiction-highly-processed-food-among-older-adults

Gessler, B., Eriksson, O., & Angenete, E. (2017). Diagnosis, treatment, and consequences of anastomotic leakage in colorectal surgery. *International Journal of Colorectal Disorders, 32*(4), 549–556.

Gill, L. E., Bartels, S. J., & Batsis, J. A. (2017). Weight management in older adults. *Current Obesity Reports, 4*(3), 379–388.

Grodstein, F., Levine, R., Troy, L., Colditz, G. A., & Stampfer, M. J. (1996). Three-year follow-up of participants in a commercial weight loss program. Can you keep it off? *Archives of International Medicine, 156*(12), 1302–1306.

Guarnotta, E. (2021, September 9). *What is a functioning alcoholic and how does it differ from an alcoholic?* GoodRx. https://www.goodrx.com/conditions/substance-use-disorder/whats-a-functioning-alcoholic

Gunners, K. (2019, July 3). *Top 12 biggest myths about weight loss.* Healthline. https://www.healthline.com/nutrition/top-12-biggest-myths-about-weight-loss

Guo, F., Bostean, G., Berardi, V., Valesquez, A. J., & Robinette, J. W. (2022). Obesogenic environments and cardiovascular disease: A path analysis using US nationally representative data. *BMC Public Health Journal 22*, 703.

Habit. (2017, September 20). *7 of the craziest fad diets of all time.* Medium. https://medium.com/habit-expert-insiders/7-of-the-craziest-fad-diets-of-all-time-bc1eda0f4893

Haden, J. (2015, November 5). *5 motivational quotes that will inspire you to believe in yourself.* Inc. Africa. https://incafrica.com/article/jeff-haden-55-motivational-quotes-which-will-inspire-you-to-believe-in-yourself

Healthier Weight. (2021, December 8). *8 celebs who had weight loss surgery.* https://www.healthierweight.co.uk/blog/celebs-who-have-had-weight-loss-surgery/

Healthy grains and how to enjoy them. (2021, December 11). Nourish by WebMD. https://www.webmd.com/diet/ss/slideshow-healthy-whole-grains

Hession, M., Rolland, C., Kulkarni, U. Wise, A., & Broom, J. (2009). Systematic review of randomized controlled trials of low-carbohydrate vs. low-fat/low-calorie diets in the management of obesity and its comorbidities. *Obesity Reviews, 10*(1), 36–50.

Hong, H.-R., Jeong, J.-O., Kong, J.-Y., Lee, S.-H., Yang, S.-H., Ha, C.-D., & Kang, H.-S. (2014). Effect of walking exercise on abdominal fat, insulin resistance and serum cytokines in obese women. *Journal of Exercise Nutrition & Biochemistry, 18*(3), 277–285.

Horikawa, C., Kodoma, S., Yatchi, Y., Heianze, Y., Hirasawa, R., Ibe, Y., Saito, K., Shimano, H., Yamada, N., & Sone, H. (2011). Skipping breakfast and prevalence of overweight and obesity in Asian and Pacific regions: A meta-analysis. *Preventive Medicine, 53*(4–5), 260–267.

Hood, M. (n.d.). *What is metabolism: Tips to increase a slow metabolism.* ShapeFit. https://www.shapefit.com/health/what-is-metabolism.html

Johns Hopkins Medicine. (n.d.). *Maintaining weight loss.* https://www.hopkinsmedicine.org/health/wellness-and-prevention/maintaining-weight-loss

Kassel, G. (2018, November 21). *Metabolism to mental health: 7 ways losing weight too fast will backfire.* Healthline. https://www.healthline.com/health/food-nutrition/rapid-weight-loss-dangers

Kennedy, S. (2021, August 18). *Big-boned, big myth.* Motion Health & Fitness. https://motionhealth.net/2021/08/18/big-boned-big-myth/

Klara, R. (2015, June 18). *Throwback Thursday: When doctors prescribed 'healthy' cigarette brands.* AdWeek. https://www.adweek.com/brand-marketing/throwback-thursday-when-doctors-prescribed-healthy-cigarette-brands-165404/#

Lean body mass explained. (2020, March 3). Tanita. https://tanita.eu/blog/lean-body-mass-explained

Lee, B.-A., & Oh, D.-J. (2015). Effect of regular swimming exercise on the physical composition, strength, and blood lipid of middle-aged women. *Journal of Exercise Rehabilitation, 11*(5), 266–271.

Lee, J. S., Jin, M. H., & Lee, H. J. (2022). Global relationship between parent and child obesity: a systematic review and meta-analysis. *Clinical and Experimental Pediatrics, 65*(1), 35–46.

Lemmer, J. T., Ivey, F. M., Ryan, A. S., Martel, G. F., Hurlbut, D. E., Metter, J. E., Fozard, J. L., Fleg, J. L., & Hurley, B. F. (2021). Effect of strength training on resting metabolic rate and physical activity: Age and gender comparisons. *Medicine & Science in Sports & Exercise, 33*(4),

532–541.

Lissner, L. Heitmann, B. (2013). Weight management: Weight cycling/weight change. In C. Caballero (ed.). *Encyclopedia of Human Nutrition* (*3rd edition*), Elsevier. https://www.sciencedirect.com/topics/agricultural-and-biological-sciences/weight-cycling

Livingstone, E. H. (2010). The incidence of bariatric surgery has plateaued in the U.S. *American Journal of Surgery, 200*(3), 378–385.

MacGill, M. (2023, January 3). *What is a normal blood pressure reading?* Medical News Today. https://www.medicalnewstoday.com/articles/270644

Mann, T., Tomiya, A. J., Westling, E., Lew, A.-M., Samuels, B., & Chatman, J. (2007). Medicare's search for effective obesity treatments: Diets are not the answer. *American Psychologist, 62*(3), 220–233.

Mayo Clinic Staff. (2021, May 6). *Metabolic syndrome.* Mayo Clinic. https://www.mayoclinic.org/diseases-conditions/metabolic-syndrome/symptoms-causes/syc-20351916

Mayo Clinic Staff. (2021, December 11). *Alcohol use: Weighing risks and benefits.* Mayo Clinic. https://www.mayoclinic.org/healthy-lifestyle/nutrition-and-healthy-eating/in-depth/alcohol/art-20044551

Mayo Clinic Staff. (2022, June 25). *Sleeve gastrectomy.* Mayo Clinic. https://www.mayoclinic.org/tests-procedures/sleeve-gastrectomy/about/pac-20385183

Mayo Clinic Staff. (2022, October 29). *Prescription weight-loss drugs.* Mayo Clinic. https://www.mayoclinic.org/healthy-lifestyle/weight-loss/in-depth/weight-loss-drugs/art-20044832

Mayo Clinic Staff. (2023, January 4) *Gastroesophageal reflux disease (GERD).* Mayo Clinic. https://www.mayoclinic.org/diseases-conditions/gerd/symptoms-causes/syc-20361940

Mayo Clinic Staff. (2023, March 13) *Type 2 diabetes.* Mayo Clinic. https://www.mayoclinic.org/diseases-conditions/type-2-diabetes/symptoms-causes/syc-20351193

Medline Plus. (n.d.). *Gastric bypass surgery.* https://medlineplus.gov/ency/article/007199.htm

Most visited cooking and recipes websites. (n.d.). Similar Web. https://www.similarweb.com/top-websites/food-and-drink/cooking-and-recipes/

Most weight lost in a lifetime (male). (n.d.). Guinness World Records. https://www.guinnessworldrecords.com/world-records/91475-most-weight-lost-in-a-lifetime-male

Nakata, Y., Okada, M., Hashimoto, K., Harada, Y., Sone, H., & Tanaka, K. (2014). Weight loss maintenance for 2 years after a 6-month randomized controlled trial comparing education-only and group-based support in Japanese adults. *Obesity Facts, 7*(6), 367–387.

National Health Service. (2022, November 28). *What is the body mass index (BMI)?* https://www.nhs.uk/common-health-questions/lifestyle/what-is-the-body-mass-index-bmi/

Newman, A. M. (2009). Obesity in older adults. *The Online Journal of Issues in Nursing, 14*(1), 03.

One in eight Americans over 50 show signs of food addiction. (2023, January 30). Science Daily. https://www.sciencedaily.com/releases/2023/01/230130090408.htm

Patterson, R. E., Frank, L. L., Kristal, A. R., & White, E. (2004). A comprehensive examination of health conditions associated with obesity in older adults. *American Journal of Preventive Medicine, 27*(5), 385–390.

Pietiläinen, K. H., Saarni, S. E., Kapiro, J., & Rissanen, A. (2012). Does dieting make you fat? A twin study. *International Journal of Obesity, 36*(3), 456–464.

Pu, C., & Syu, H.-F. (2023). Effects of disability on income and income composition. *PloS One, 18*(5).

Raman, M. (2023, February 23). *The 8 best exercises for weight loss.* Healthline. https://www.healthline.com/nutrition/best-exercise-for-weight-loss

Raman, R. (2023, June 23). *Is it bad to lose weight too quickly?* Healthline. https://www.healthline.com/nutrition/losing-weight-too-fast

Ravelli, G. P., Stein, Z. A., & Susser, M. W. (1976). Obesity in young men after famine exposure in utero and early infancy. *New England Journal of Medicine, 295*(7), 349–352.

Roberts, S. B., & Das, S. K. (2017, June 1). *Want to lose weight? What you need to know about eating and exercise.* Scientific American. https://www.scientificamerican.com/article/want-to-lose-weight-what-you-need-to-know-about-eating-and-exercise/

Schuit, A. J., van Loon, A. J. M., Tijhuis, M., & Ocké, MC. (2002). Clustering of lifestyle risk factors in a general adult population. *Preventive Medicine Journal, 35*(3), 219–224.

Seaver, V. (2023, July 11). *7-day heart-healthy meal plan: 1,200 calories.* Eating Well. https://www.eatingwell.com/article/289245/7-day-heart-healthy-meal-plan-1200-calories/

Seddon, M. (2012, March 16). *A Staten Island man's heartbreaking battle with obesity.* SILive. https://www.silive.com/news/2012/03/a_staten_island_mans_heartbrea.html

Simon, G. E., Von Korff, M., Saunders, K., Miglioretti, D. L., Crane, P. K., van Belle, G., & Kessler, R. C. (2006). Association between obesity and psychiatric disorders in the U.S. adult population. *Archives of General Psychiatry, 63*(7), 824–830.

Spritzler, F. (2020, March 9). *Do 'diets' really just make you fatter?* Healthline. https://www.healthline.com/nutrition/do-diets-make-you-gain-weight

Stanner, S. A., Bulmer, K., Andrès, K., Lantseva, O. E., Borodina, V., Poteen, V. V., & Yudkin, J. S. (1997). Does malnutrition in utero determine diabetes and coronary heart disease in adulthood? Results from the Leningrad Siege study, a cross sectional study. *BMJ, 315*(7119), 1342–1348.

Student found dead after going on extreme diet to lose weight for upcoming holiday, inquest hears. (2019, October 29). *The Telegraph.* https://www.telegraph.co.uk/news/2019/10/29/student-found-dead-going-extreme-diet-lose-weight-upcoming-holiday/

Suni, E., & Singh, A. (2023, March 22). *How much sleep do we really need?* Sleep Foundation. https://www.sleepfoundation.org/how-sleep-works/how-much-sleep-do-we-really-need

Swinburn, B., Egger, G., & Raza, F. (1999). Dissecting obesogenic environments: The development and application of a framework for identifying and prioritizing environmental interventions for obesity. *Journal of Preventive Medicine, 29*(6 Pt 1), 563–570.

10 secrets for balanced whole-body wellness. (2018, February 22). Sarasota Smile Design. https://www.sarasotasmiledesign.com/10-secrets-balanced-whole-body-wellness/

Vafiadis, D. (2021, April 21). *How excess weight impacts our mental and emotional health.* National Council on Aging. https://www.ncoa.org/

article/how-excess-weight-impacts-our-mental-and-emotional-health

Vink, R. G., Roumans, N. J. T., Arkenbosch, L. A. J., Mariman, E. C. M., & van Baak, M. A. (2016). The effect of rate of weight loss on long-term weight regain in adults with overweight and obesity. *Obesity, 24*(2), 321–327.

A visual guide to heart disease. (2021, June 30). WebMD. https://www. webmd.com/heart-disease/ss/slideshow-visual-guide-to-heart-disease

Waehner, P. (2020, November 9). *Seated total body workout for overweight exercisers.* Verywell Fit. https://www.verywellfit.com/seated-total-body-for-overweight-and-obese-exercisers-1231355

Wannamethee, S. G., Shaper, A. G., & Walker, M. (2001). Weight change, body weight and mortality: The impact of smoking and ill health. *International Journal of Epidemiology, 30*(4), 777–786.

Ward, Z. J., Willett, W. C., Hu, F. B., Pacheco, L. S., Long, M. W., & Gortmaker, S. L. (2022). Excess mortality associated with elevated body weight in the USA by state and demographic subgroup: A modeling study. *eClinicalMedicine, 48,* 101429.

WebMD Editorial Contributors. (2021, June 22). *What is metabolism?* WebMD. https://www.webmd.com/fitness-exercise/what-is-metabolism

WebMD Editorial Contributors (2021, November 13). *How to measure your waist.* WebMD. https://www.webmd.com/diet/guide/calculating-your-waist-circumference

What is fartlek training? (n.d.). Asics. https://www.asics.com/gb/en-gb/running-advice/what-is-fartlek-training

What is weight management and why is it important? (n.d.). Southside Medical. https://southsidemedical.net/what-is-weight-management-and-why-is-it-important/

Whitaker, R. C., Pepe, M. S., Wright, J. A., Seidal, K. D., & Dietz, W. H. (1998). Early adiposity rebound and the risk of adult obesity. *Pediatrics, 101*(3), E5.

Wilding, J. P. H. (2014). The importance of weight management in type 2 diabetes mellitus. *International Journal of Clinical Practice, 68*(6), 682–691.

Woźniewska, P., Diemieszczyk, I., & Hady, H. R. (2021). Complications associated with laparoscopic sleeve gastrectomy: A review. *Przeglad Gastroenterologiczny, 16*(1), 5–9.

Yan, L. L, Daviglus, M. L., Liu, K., Pirzada, A., Garside, D. B., Schiffer, L., Dyer, A. R., &Greenland, P. (2004). BMI and health-related quality of life in adults 65 years and older. *Obesity Research & Clinical Practice, 12,* 69–76.

IMAGE REFERENCES

Andres, A. (2021, January 20). *Green apple with measuring tape on table in kitchen* [Image]. Pexels. https://www.pexels.com/photo/green-apple-with-measuring-tape-on-table-in-kitchen-6550823/

Ann, H. (2019, October 17). *No smoking sign* [Image]. Pexels. https://www.pexels.com/photo/no-smoking-sign-3095752/

Ann, H. (2019, July 11). *Start written on asphalt.* [Image]. Pexels. https://www.pexels.com/photo/start-written-on-asphalt-2646531/

Ayrton, A. (2021, January 20). *Woman showing apple and bitten doughnut* [Image]. Pexels. https://www.pexels.com/photo/woman-showing-apple-and-bitten-doughnut-6551415/

Barbhuiya, T. (2021, October 17). *A person holding his belly fat* [Image]. Pexels. https://www.pexels.com/photo/a-person-holding-his-belly-fat-9927899/

Borba, J. (2019, October 14). *Woman holding two ropes in gym* [Image]. Pexels. https://www.pexels.com/photo/woman-holding-two-ropes-in-gym-3076511/

Cottonbro. (2020, June 29). *Man in black pants and black tank top standing on wooden floor.* [Image]. Pexels. https://www.pexels.com/photo/man-in-black-pants-and-black-tank-top-standing-on-brown-wooden-floor-4752861/

Filkins, A. (2020, October 9). *Cute black girl in chef costume* [Image]. Pexels. https://www.pexels.com/photo/cute-black-girl-in-chef-costume-5561131/

Green, A. (2020, October 25). *Little girl eating huge delicious sandwich*

[Image]. Pexels. https://www.pexels.com/photo/little-girl-eating-huge-delicious-sandwich-5693056/

Katyal, P. (2019, August 1). *Close-up photography of a cell phone* [Image]. Pexels. https://www.pexels.com/photo/close-up-photography-of-a-cellphone-2740955/

Magners, M. (2021, February 1). *Woman holding a blue paper with message* [Image]. Pexels. https://www.pexels.com/photo/woman-carrying-a-blue-paper-with-message-6670508/

Miroshnichenko, T. (2021, January 3). *Man doing crossfit* [Image]. Pexels. https://www.pexels.com/photo/man-doing-crossfit-6389075/

Oquendo, C. (2019, October 8). *Man wearing black blazer* [Image]. Pexels. https://www.pexels.com/photo/man-wearing-black-blazer-3051576/

Piacquadio, A. (2020, February 20). *Happy diverse sportspeople jogging in park* [Image]. Pexels. https://www.pexels.com/photo/happy-diverse-sportspeople-jogging-in-park-3776816/

Piacquadio, A. (2020, February 19). *Sportive woman with bicycle resting on countryside road in sunlight.* [Image]. Pexels. https://www.pexels.com/photo/sportive-woman-with-bicycle-resting-on-countryside-road-in-sunlight-3771836/

Piacquadio, A. (2020, February 18). *Young athletes preparing for running in training hall* [Image]. Pexels. https://www.pexels.com/photo/young-athletes-preparing-for-running-in-training-hall-3764014/

Pixabay. (2017, July 20). *Green Apple Fruit.* [Image]. Pexels. https://www.pexels.com/photo/green-apple-fruit-533343/

RUN 4 FFWPU. (2018, November 1). *Man running on black asphalt road* [Image]. Pexels. https://www.pexels.com/photo/man-running-on-black-asphalt-road-1555354/

Schvets, A. (2020, March 2). *Medical equipment on an operating room* [Image]. Pexels. https://www.pexels.com/photo/medical-equipment-on-an-operation-room-3844581/

Shivers. (2021, February 27). *Woman weighing on scales in studio* [Image]. Pexels. https://www.pexels.com/photo/woman-weighing-on-scales-in-studio-6975474/

Snapwire. (2017, October 17). *People doing marathon* [Image]. Pexels. https://www.pexels.com/photo/people-doing-marathon-618612/

Souza, S. (2019, February 22). *Aerial ocean shot* [Image]. Pexels. https://www.pexels.com/photo/aerial-ocean-shot-1936954/1